D0673845

a simple guide to
cholesterol

BESTMEDICINE Health Handbooks

A Simple Guide to Cholesterol
First published – September 2005

Published by
CSF Medical Communications Ltd
1 Bankside, Lodge Road, Long Hanborough
Oxfordshire, OX29 8LJ, UK
T +44 (0)1993 885370 F +44 (0)1993 881868
enquiries@bestmedicine.com
www.bestmedicine.com
www.csfmedical.com

Editor Dr Eleanor Bull
Medical Editor Dr Jonathan Morrell
Creative Director & Project Manager Julia Potterton
Designer Lee Smith
Layout Julie Smith
Publisher Stephen I'Anson

ISBN: 1-905466-05-6

BESTMEDICINE is a trademark of CSF Medical Communications Ltd

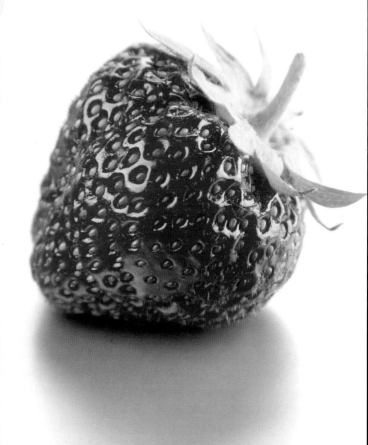

contents

ACKNOWLEDGEMENTS

The *BESTMEDICINE Simple Guides* team is very grateful to a number of people who have made this project possible. In particular we'd like to thank Anne Taylor, Jane Cassidy, Caroline Delasalle and Amelie (5 months). Thank you to Ben for his endless enthusiasm, energy and creativity, to Molly (7) and George (5) and of course to Hetta. Julie and Rob who went far beyond the call of duty and Julie's ability to put pages together for hours on end was hugely inspiring. Thanks also to Jacqui Morrell for reviewing the manuscript.

A Simple Guide to your Health Service

Emma Catherall   Co-ordinator

Advisory Panel

Richard Stevens   GP
Anne Taylor   Practice nurse
Julie Lovegrove   Dietitian
Michael Gum   Pharmacist
John Chater   Binley's health and care
                     information specialist
                     www.binleys.com

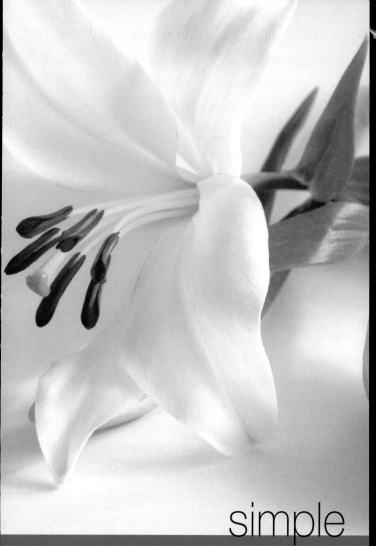

simple

simple *adj.* **1.** easy to understand or do: *a simple problem.* **2.** plain; unadorned: *a simple dress.* **3.** Not combined or complex: *a simple mechanism.* **4.** Unaffected or unpretentious: *although he became famous he remained a simple man.* **5.** sincere; frank: *a simple explanation was readily accepted.* **6.** (*prenominal*) without additions or modifications: *the witness told the simple truth.*

ABOUT THE AUTHOR

ELEANOR BULL

Eleanor graduated from King's College London with a BSc Honours degree in Pharmacology and then completed a PhD in Neuroscience at the University of Nottingham. As well as publishing her own research work internationally, Eleanor has written for numerous publications in the BESTMEDICINE series. She now lives in the West of Ireland.

ABOUT THE EDITOR

JONATHAN MORRELL

Jonathan Morrell is a practising GP and a hospital practitioner in cardiology. He was a founding trustee and director of HEART UK (Hyperlipidaemia Education And Research Trust) and is also a member of the British Cardiac Society.

FOREWORD

TRISHA MACNAIR

Doctor and BBC Health Journalist

Getting involved in managing your own medical condition – or helping those you love or care for to manage theirs – is a vital step towards keeping as healthy as possible. Whilst doctors, nurses and the rest of your healthcare team can help you with expert advice and guidance, nobody knows your body, your symptoms and what is right for *you* as well as you do.

There is no long-term (chronic) medical condition or illness that I can think of where the person concerned has absolutely no influence at all on their situation. The way you choose to live your life, from the food you eat to the exercise you take, will impact upon your disease, your well-being and how able you are to cope. You are in charge!

Being involved in making choices about your treatment helps you to feel in control of your problems, and makes sure you get the help that you really need. Research clearly shows that when people living with a chronic illness take an active role in looking after themselves, they can bring about significant improvements in their illness and vastly improve the quality of life they enjoy. Of course, there may be occasions when you feel particularly unwell and it all seems out of your control. Yet most of the time there are plenty of things that you can do in order to reduce the negative effects that your condition can have on your life. This way you feel as good as possible and may even be able to alter the course of your condition.

So how do you gain the confidence and skills to take an active part in managing your condition, communicate with health professionals and work through sometimes worrying and emotive issues? The answer is to become better informed. Reading about your problem, talking to others who have been through similar experiences and hearing what the experts have to say will all help to build-up your understanding and help you to take an active role in your own health care.

BESTMEDICINE Simple Guides provide an invaluable source of help, giving you the facts that you need in order to understand the key issues and discuss them with your doctors and other professionals involved in your care. The information is presented in an accessible way but without neglecting the important details. Produced independently and under the guidance of medical experts *A Simple Guide to Cholesterol* is an evidence-based, balanced and up-to-date review that I hope you will find enables you to play an active part in the successful management of your condition.

what happens normally?

WHAT HAPPENS NORMALLY?

Cholesterol is a fatty substance that is made by the liver. It can be found all over our bodies and plays an important role in our day-to-day functioning.

WHAT IS CHOLESTEROL EXACTLY?

Humans have an estimated 100,000 billion cells.

Cholesterol is a soft, fatty substance found in every cell of our bodies.

WHERE DOES IT COME FROM?

There are two ways in which we acquire cholesterol.
1. We make it ourselves in our liver.
2. We get it from the food we eat.

Contrary to popular opinion, our liver makes most of the cholesterol we have in our bodies, with only a small proportion coming directly from our diet. Foods that are rich in cholesterol include dairy produce, fatty meats, egg yolks, offal and seafood (especially shellfish). Plant-derived foods contain no cholesterol. The body can be pretty good at balancing the cholesterol we make with the cholesterol we get from our food; the more cholesterol-rich food we eat, the less the body ought to make. However, if our diet is high in saturated fat then our cholesterol levels can become unbalanced. This has the potential to cause serious problems to our health and can even be fatal if left unchecked.

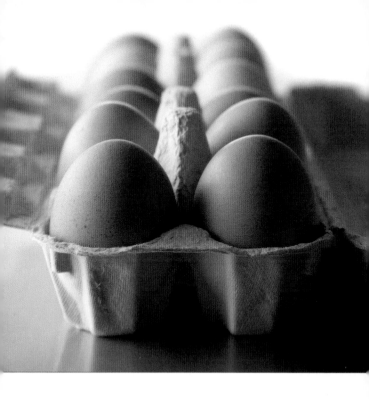

WHY DO WE NEED CHOLESTEROL?

Cholesterol plays a vital role in the day-to-day
functioning of our bodies. Put simply, without
cholesterol we could not survive. Apart from
anything else, cholesterol forms a major part
of the outer perimeter, or membrane, of every
cell in our bodies and helps to control which
substances can enter or leave a cell. We also
need it to:

- make certain hormones
- make certain vitamins
- ensure our digestive system works properly
  by helping to form bile.

Bile is a greenish
brown fluid that is
essential for the
digestion of food.

3

THE CHOLESTEROL TRANSPORT SYSTEM

Lipoproteins are transporters that carry fats and fat-like substances (such as cholesterol) in the blood.

Cholesterol cannot travel around the body on its own because it won't dissolve in water. So instead, it is transported as part of structures called lipoproteins. Think of lipoproteins as lorries that transport cholesterol around the body. There are many different types of lipoprotein, but the two major kinds that we need to think about are:

■ low density lipoprotein (LDL)
■ high density lipoprotein (HDL).

Cholesterol itself is always the same. It is the carrier vehicle, the 'lorry', or lipoprotein it is attached to that determines what happens to the cholesterol it is carrying.

■ LDL cholesterol transports cholesterol from where it is made in the liver to the tissues of the body that need it. LDL is the major cholesterol transporter in the blood.
■ HDL cholesterol removes excess cholesterol from the tissues and brings it back to the liver for reprocessing or removal from the body altogether.

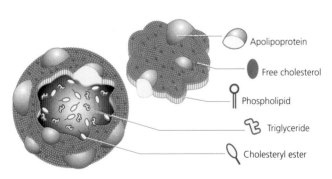

Apolipoprotein

Free cholesterol

Phospholipid

Triglyceride

Cholesteryl ester

THE STRUCTURE OF A LIPOPROTEIN.

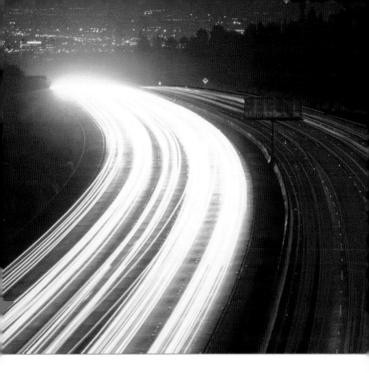

The levels of substances called triglycerides in our bloodstream are often grouped together with our levels of cholesterol. Triglycerides are fats that are found in meat, dairy produce and cooking oils and are a major source of energy for body tissues. They are also found in the fat stores of our bodies and are made from scratch in the liver. Like cholesterol, triglycerides are fats that circulate in your blood. Collectively, LDL and HDL cholesterol and triglycerides are known as 'blood lipids'.

'Blood lipids' is the collective term for all of the fatty substances found in the blood. It includes LDL and HDL cholesterol and triglycerides.

5

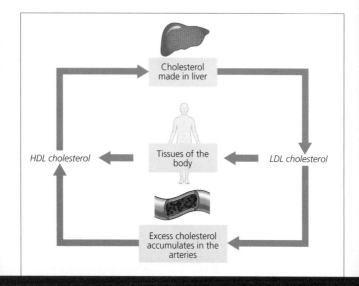

LDL *cholesterol transports cholesterol from the liver to the tissues of the body and HDL cholesterol removes excess cholesterol from the tissues and brings it back to the liver. As a general rule, HDL cholesterol is 'the good guy' and LDL cholesterol and triglycerides are 'the bad guys'. We will explain why and what we can do to raise HDL and lower LDL cholesterol in the next sections of* A Simple Guide to Cholesterol.

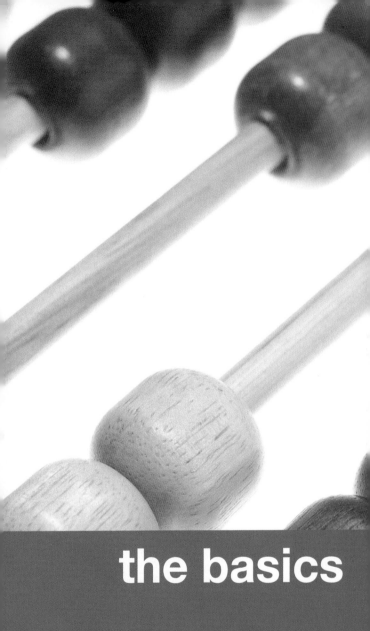

the basics

CHOLESTEROL – THE BASICS

If the levels of the different types of cholesterol in our bloodstream become abnormal, they can start to affect how well our heart and circulation works. This is why it is so important that we are aware of our cholesterol levels and take steps to control them.

Our heart pumps about 7,000 litres of blood through our circulatory system every day.

Your circulatory system comprises your heart and the vast network of arteries and veins that carry your blood around the body to where it is needed. Maintaining a healthy circulation is key to enjoying a long and active life. If our circulation is compromised or restricted in any way, the part of the body or the organ that it supplies are no longer able to function properly, and this can have devastating consequences for our health and well-being.

In the previous section we explained that our total blood cholesterol includes two major components, HDL ('good' cholesterol) and LDL ('bad' cholesterol). If LDL cholesterol is too high and HDL cholesterol too low, then our chances of developing heart and other circulatory (or 'vascular') diseases (known collectively as cardiovascular diseases) can increase. In addition, raised levels of triglycerides (which are often found with low levels of HDL cholesterol) are dangerous in themselves and also have the effect of making LDL cholesterol more damaging and HDL cholesterol less protective.

The term 'dyslipidaemia' describes abnormal blood lipid (fat) levels. This includes abnormal levels of LDL and HDL cholesterol, as well as triglycerides.

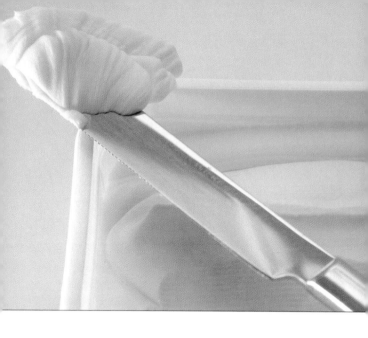

THE DIFFERENCE BETWEEN 'BAD' AND 'GOOD'

Having high cholesterol is not always a bad thing. Having high levels of 'good' HDL cholesterol can help to keep our arteries healthy. This is why the term 'high cholesterol' can sometimes be misleading.

It is both the levels and the balance of the various lipids in our blood that determines how healthy our circulation is.

Strictly speaking, it is more accurate to talk about 'abnormal lipids' than it is to talk about 'high cholesterol'. 'Lipids' is the collective term for all of the fatty substances that are found in the blood. It includes LDL and HDL cholesterol and triglycerides (the fats found in meat, dairy produce and cooking oils). It's a common misconception. Many of us, including some doctors, still refer to 'high cholesterol'. Using this term is all very well, providing you remember that 'high' cholesterol per se may not tell the full story.

BALANCING THE NUMBERS

After you have had your cholesterol measured, the number you will be given usually refers to the **total** amount of cholesterol in your bloodstream at a particular point in time (e.g. 'you have a cholesterol of 5.8'). Cholesterol is measured as millimoles of cholesterol per litre of blood plasma or serum, shortened to mmol/L.

In the UK, your total cholesterol is considered to be high if it exceeds 5 (or 5 mmol/L). The number has come down over the years as the results of clinical trials involving many thousands of patients have confirmed that the lower your cholesterol, the longer you live. Simple as that!

As mentioned previously, the relative levels of 'bad' LDL and 'good' HDL cholesterol are also important. If your cholesterol is above 5 but you have a high level of HDL cholesterol, your doctor will not be as concerned as they would if you had a high level of LDL cholesterol. It is recommended that your levels of LDL cholesterol do not exceed 3 mmol/L.

WHY IS LDL CHOLESTEROL BAD?

If too much LDL cholesterol is circulating in our bloodstream, over time it slowly builds up in the inner walls of the arteries that supply the organs of the body with the oxygen and nutrients they need. This build-up of LDL cholesterol can narrow and clog our arteries with something called atheroma. The process itself is known as atherosclerosis.

Atherosclerosis can restrict our blood flow so much that the amount of oxygen it supplies to the various organs of the body falls below the amount needed to function properly.

This can mean that there are times when our circulation just can't supply the extra oxygen we need (for example when we are exercising). This lack of oxygen can affect our legs when we run or walk, and can cause heart pain or 'angina'. These warning pains will normally go away when we rest, but should a vital artery become completely clogged then the muscle being supplied will die from oxygen starvation. If the muscle in question is our heart, we experience a potentially fatal heart attack.

THE 'H' IN HDL STANDS FOR 'HEALTHY'

In contrast to LDL cholesterol, HDL cholesterol carries excess cholesterol away from artery walls and back to the liver, where it is removed from the body as bile which exits the body in our faeces. This is why HDL is the good guy, because it helps to clear up excess cholesterol from the body and so slows the development of atherosclerosis, protecting us against heart and other vascular diseases. As well as standing for 'healthy' the 'H' in HDL could also stand for 'hoover'!

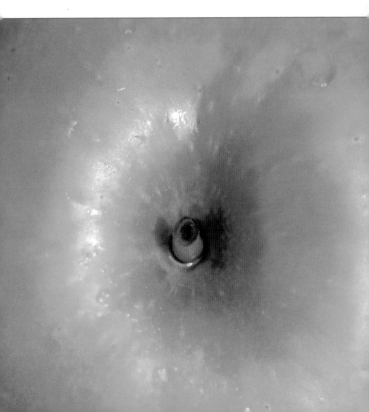

THE TRIGLYCERIDE CONNECTION

Just to complicate matters, triglycerides are another potential 'bad guy' that we need to be aware of. Like LDL cholesterol, high blood levels of triglycerides are associated with an increased risk of developing heart and other vascular diseases. People with high triglycerides (currently considered to be anything above 1.7 mmol/L), often have high total cholesterol, high LDL cholesterol and low HDL cholesterol. The triple whammy! Although high triglycerides have some risk in their own right, they are especially risky when present with low levels of HDL cholesterol, a situation that is often seen in people with diabetes or pre-diabetes. Raised triglycerides also make LDL cholesterol more toxic and dangerous to artery linings (making 'bad' cholesterol 'worse') and reduce the beneficial effects of 'good' HDL cholesterol.

All of the fatty substances found in our blood including LDL and HDL cholesterol and triglycerides are referred to as blood lipids.

LDL cholesterol – the LOWER the better.
HDL cholesterol – the HIGHER the better.

WHAT UPSETS OUR CHOLESTEROL BALANCE?

There are a number of reasons why our cholesterol levels can become abnormal and affect our health. Having too much saturated fat in our diet is an obvious cause that we can all do something about. We will look at strategies to help you achieve a healthy diet later on in this book.

Raised cholesterol is to some extent an unavoidable part of getting older. Or to look at it another way, the older you are, the more time you have had to do damage to your body! Not exercising enough can damage our health in many ways, and not just by causing us to gain weight. The benefits of exercise have knock-on effects on many other aspects

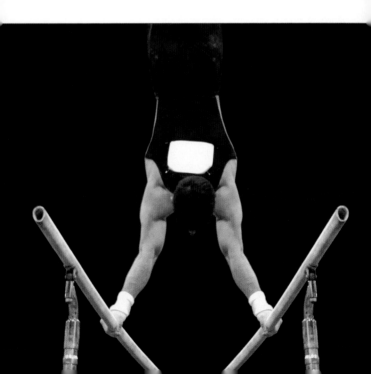

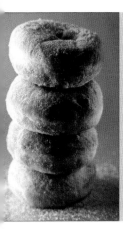

WHY IS MY LDL CHOLESTEROL TOO HIGH?

Common reasons include:
- advancing age
- your gender
- your genetic/ethnic make-up
- having a poor diet (specifically eating too much saturated fat) and being overweight
- a lack of physical activity
- having diabetes.

of cardiovascular health, cholesterol being one of these. Regular exercise can increase levels of 'good' HDL cholesterol.

Unfortunately, some people cannot help having lipid problems because they were born with them. One of the medical conditions in which high levels of LDL cholesterol are inherited is called familial hypercholesterolaemia.

FAMILIAL HYPERCHOLESTEROLAEMIA (FH)

About 1 in 500 people in the UK have familial hypercholesterolaemia. This is an inherited disorder and is about as common as insulin dependent (or type 1) diabetes. The inheritance of familial hypercholesterolaemia is 50/50 meaning that in the same way that the disorder was passed to you from one of your parents, if you or your partner has familial hypercholesterolaemia then your child has a 50/50 chance of having it as well.

In people with familial hypercholesterolaemia, the mechanism by which LDL cholesterol is removed from the circulation works less effectively than normal. This means that their blood cholesterol level is roughly double or treble what it should be.

The abnormally high levels of cholesterol in individuals affected with familial hypercholesterolaemia can lead to premature vascular events like heart attacks and strokes. If you have a family history of these problems talk to your doctor or health practitioner and arrange to have your cholesterol checked. There are treatments available today that can significantly reduce your risk of the associated cardiovascular diseases even if you have familial hypercholesterolaemia. The important thing is to find out about it as soon as you can by talking to your doctor, practice nurse or pharmacist, and by having your cholesterol checked.

CARDIOVASCULAR DISEASE AND LIPID DISORDERS

Cardiovascular disease (CVD) is an umbrella term that is used to describe medical conditions that affect the heart and the circulatory system (arteries and veins).

Having high cholesterol or abnormal lipids can be harmful because they increase your chances of developing some types of cardiovascular disease, diseases that affect the heart and the circulatory system. The term coronary heart disease describes two of the most common conditions – heart attack and angina – that occur as a result of having high cholesterol or abnormal lipids.

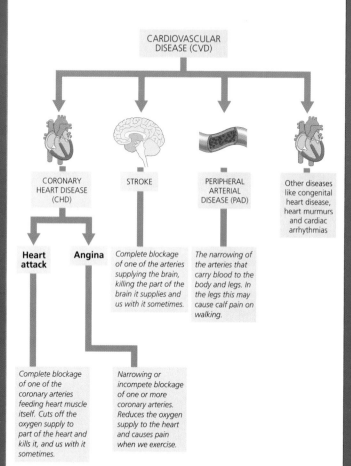

CARDIOVASCULAR
DISEASE (CVD)

CORONARY
HEART DISEASE
(CHD)

STROKE

PERIPHERAL
ARTERIAL
DISEASE (PAD)

Other diseases
like congenital
heart disease,
heart murmurs
and cardiac
arrhythmias

Heart attack

Angina

*Complete blockage
of one of the arteries
supplying the brain,
killing the part of the
brain it supplies and
us with it sometimes.*

*The narrowing of
the arteries that
carry blood to the
body and legs. In
the legs this may
cause calf pain on
walking.*

*Complete blockage
of one of the
coronary arteries
feeding heart muscle
itself. Cuts off the
oxygen supply to
part of the heart and
kills it, and us with it
sometimes.*

*Narrowing or
incompete blockage
of one or more
coronary arteries.
Reduces the oxygen
supply to the heart
and causes pain
when we exercise.*

ATHEROSCLEROSIS

For many types of cardiovascular condition; the underlying cause is atherosclerosis. This describes the process by which the lining of your artery walls becomes furred with a thick sludge-like substance (called atheroma) made up of fatty deposits of cholesterol and other substances. Much like the limescale furring of a water pipe, unless action is taken, atherosclerosis will continue until the entire artery (or pipe) becomes blocked and no blood (or water) can flow through it. Often the blood becomes more prone to clotting. This is when the health problems really start.

A fragile atheromatous deposit can potentially split open exposing its contents to the bloodstream. In an effort to repair this damage a blood clot will form which may

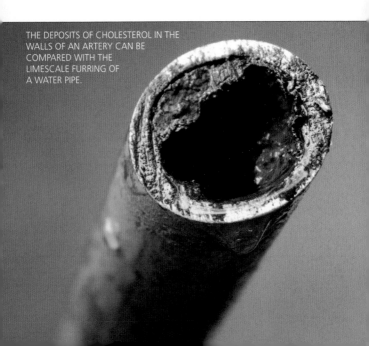

THE DEPOSITS OF CHOLESTEROL IN THE WALLS OF AN ARTERY CAN BE COMPARED WITH THE LIMESCALE FURRING OF A WATER PIPE.

ATHEROSCLEROSIS CAN LEAD TO:
- heart attacks (myocardial infarction)
- angina
- stroke
- peripheral arterial disease (PAD; affects the aorta and leg arteries).

completely block the artery concerned and lead to an emergency situation.

If the blockage occurs in the arteries that supply your heart then this can cause a heart attack or angina (a pain that tells us our heart is not receiving enough oxygen). If the affected arteries are those of the brain then this can cause a stroke and if blood supply to the arms or legs is reduced, it can cause difficulty walking and eventually gangrene (peripheral arterial disease).

The aorta is the main artery that carries blood away from the heart.

AM I AT RISK FROM CARDIOVASCULAR DISEASE?

A risk factor is anything that increases your odds of developing a disease.

Although you won't automatically develop cardiovascular disease just because you have abnormal levels of lipids in your bloodstream, the facts remain that the higher your LDL cholesterol and the lower your HDL cholesterol, the higher your risk of developing cardiovascular disease.

There are a number of other factors that can also increase your risk of developing cardiovascular disease. These include:

- smoking
- being overweight
- not doing enough exercise
- having high blood pressure
- having diabetes.

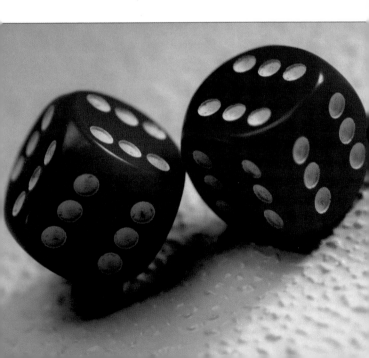

It is important to tackle these 'modifiable' risk factors because unfortunately, there are some risk factors that you can't do anything about. These are:

- having a strong history of cardiovascular disease in your family
- having pre-existing atherosclerotic disease (heart attack, angina, stroke, PAD)
- gender (cardiovascular disease is more common in men than women until older age, when it evens out)
- advancing age
- ethnic origin (people of Indo-Asian ethnicity are more at risk from cardiovascular disease).

The more of these risk factors you have, the more likely you are to develop cardiovascular disease. Because it is so common, preventing heart disease is a top priority. The good news is that this can be done by making a few changes to the way you live. We will discuss these lifestyle measures later on in the book.

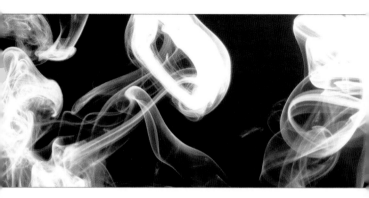

HOW WILL I KNOW IF MY CHOLESTEROL IS ABNORMAL?

Ideally, your total cholesterol level should be less than 5 mmol/L.

High cholesterol (or an abnormal lipid profile) does not usually have any noticeable symptoms. This can make it difficult to tell whether or not you are at risk. Your lipid profile can be confirmed with a simple blood test, but the difficulty is knowing whether or not to have one in the first place. There are four main reasons why you may undergo a cholesterol test.

- You may be offered a cholesterol test as part of a general check on your health to assess your cardiovascular risk (opportunistic screening).
- You may be advised to have your cholesterol checked because you have other cardiovascular risk factors or have had a cardiovascular event.
- You display signs of dyslipidaemia (e.g. cholesterol deposits on eyelids or on tendons).
- You may have a relative who has recently been diagnosed with high cholesterol.

The cholesterol test itself is very straightforward. Your doctor (or the healthcare professional doing the test) will take a blood sample from a vein in your arm using a needle. The sample is then sent off to a laboratory for analysis. Alternatively, your doctor, nurse or pharmacist may take a smaller blood sample from your finger tip and examine it on the spot using a desk-top analyser (although some of

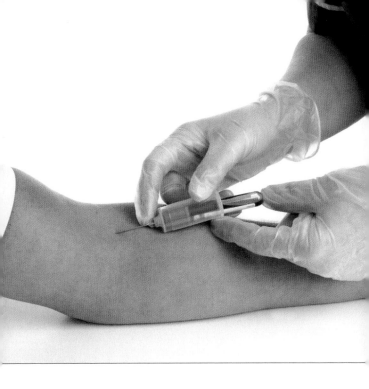

these devices can only measure total
cholesterol and not the relative proportions of
LDL and HDL cholesterol). These days there are
also a number of self-testing cholesterol kits
that can be purchased from pharmacies. Whilst
testing your own cholesterol may be more
convenient than visiting your doctor, remember
that the results may not be as accurate and
you may need professional help to work out
what they mean and what, if anything, you
should do about them. Your GP, practice nurse
and pharmacist are on hand free of charge.
Use them!

If you are having your
triglycerides measured
as part of your lipid
profile, you will be
asked to fast for
12–14 hours before
the blood test.

MANAGING CHOLESTEROL

The Joint British Societies publish national advice for health professionals and they include the British Cardiac Society, HEART UK, the British Hypertension Society, Diabetes UK and the Primary Care Cardiovascular Society.

Once you have been diagnosed with abnormal lipids, your doctor will discuss with you what this actually means. They will mention target lipid levels (as set out by national guidelines), and will discuss the best way that you can work together to achieve these targets. The overriding aim of any cholesterol management plan is to lower your cardiovascular risk and stop you from having a heart attack or stroke or suffering any other of the many cardiovascular consequences. Once you have it under control your lipid profile is something that you will have to keep an eye on for the rest of your life.

Your doctor will:
- decide whether your cholesterol is abnormal
- take into account your age, family history and other cardiovascular risk factors like your blood pressure, smoking history or whether you have diabetes.
- estimate your risk of developing cardiovascular disease in the next 10 years
- discuss and agree with you the best way to tackle the problem.

In general, there are two complementary ways to manage cholesterol:
1. making lifestyle changes (which include following a cholesterol-lowering and healthy heart diet, increasing your levels of physical activity and stopping smoking)
2. taking cholesterol-lowering drugs (as well as making the lifestyle changes listed above).

Lifestyle changes that can help to lower cholesterol and reduce cardiovascular risk

- ■ Eating less saturated fat.
- ■ Eating more fruit and vegetables.
- ■ Eating less salt.
- ■ Losing weight if you are overweight.
- ■ Being more physically active.
- ■ Giving up smoking.
- ■ Drinking alcohol in moderation.

The higher your risk of cardiovascular disease, the more likely it is that your doctor will recommend that you take medications that have been shown to lower cholesterol and help people to achieve their cholesterol targets. There are a number of drug types currently available that work in different ways. The statins are usually the first choice of treatment because of massive evidence that they work and in addition to lowering your cholesterol they may also protect your heart in other ways (such as keeping the lining of the blood vessels healthy). One statin drug, simvastatin (Zocor Heart-Pro®), is available as a low-dose tablet from your pharmacist without a prescription.

THE DIFFERENT TYPES OF CHOLESTEROL-LOWERING DRUGS

Drug type	Generic name	Brand name(s)
Statins	Atorvastatin	Lipitor®
	Fluvastatin	Lescol®
	Pravastatin	Lipostat® (plus generics)
	Rosuvastatin	Crestor®
	Simvastatin	Zocor®, Zocor Heart-Pro® (plus generics)
Fibrates	Bezafibrate	Bezalip®, Bezalip® Mono, Zimbacol®
	Ciprofibrate	Modalim®
	Fenofibrate	Lipantil®, Fenogal®, Supralip 160®
	Gemfibrozil	Lopid®
Resins	Colestyramine	Questran®, Questran Light®
	Colestipol	Colestid®
Selective cholesterol absorption inhibitors	Ezetimibe	Ezetrol®
Nicotinic acid derivatives	Nicotinic acid/niacin	Niaspan®
	Acipimox	Olbetam®
Omega-3-fish oils		Omacor®
		Maxepa®
Combination drugs	Simvastatin *plus* ezetimibe	Inegy®

Drugs often have more than one name. A generic name, which refers to its active ingredient, and a brand name, which is the registered trade name given to it by the pharmaceutical company. Simvastatin is a generic name and Zocor Heart-Pro® is a brand name.

TERMINOLOGY

Cholesterol – A soft, fatty substance found in every cell of our bodies.

LDL cholesterol (low density lipoprotein cholesterol) – Excess LDL cholesterol can build-up in the walls of arteries and can narrow and eventually clog them (a process known as atherosclerosis). LDL cholesterol is also known as 'bad' cholesterol. A high amount of LDL cholesterol in the blood is a major risk factor for cardiovascular disease.

HDL cholesterol (high density lipoprotein cholesterol) – Helps to clear up excess cholesterol from the body and hence slows the development of atherosclerosis. HDL cholesterol is also known as 'good' cholesterol. A high amount of HDL cholesterol in the blood may help to protect us against cardiovascular disease.

Cardiovascular diseases – Medical conditions that affect the heart and the circulatory system.

Hypercholesterolaemia – Excessively high levels of cholesterol in the blood.

Lipids – Fatty substances (includes LDL cholesterol, HDL cholesterol and triglycerides).

Abnormal lipids – Usually denotes high levels of LDL cholesterol and/or triglycerides or low levels of HDL cholesterol in the blood.

Dyslipidaemia – Abnormal levels of lipids or lipoproteins in the blood. This includes abnormal levels of LDL and HDL cholesterol, as well as triglycerides.

Hyperlipidaemia – Excessively high levels of lipids in the blood. This usually means high levels of LDL cholesterol and/or triglycerides.

Lipid profile – A collective term for the main fatty substances measured in the blood. Includes levels of total cholesterol, HDL cholesterol and triglycerides. In most cases, the level of LDL cholesterol can be calculated from these values.

Triglycerides – Fats that are found in meat, dairy produce and cooking oils, and produced by the body itself. Represent a major source of energy for the tissues of the body.

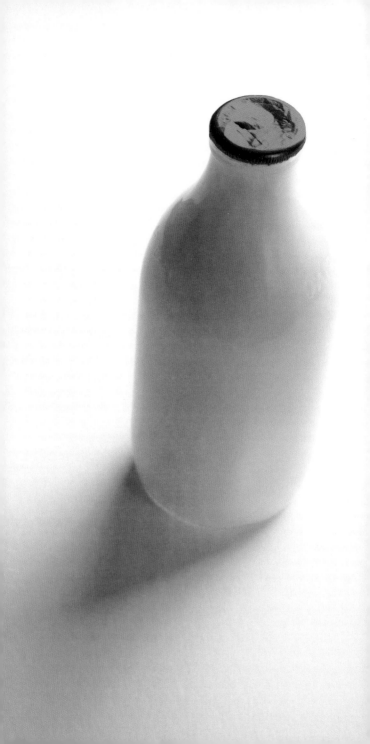

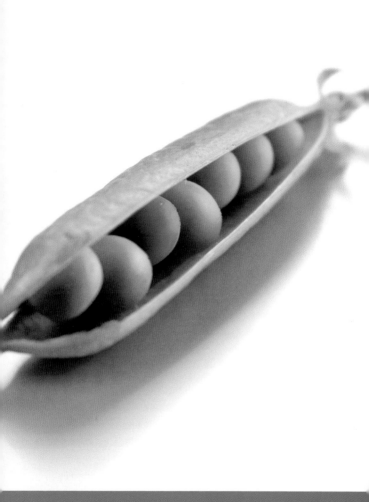

why me?

WHY ME?

If you, or a member of your family, have recently been diagnosed with high cholesterol or an unhealthy lipid profile, you are by no means alone. It is estimated that in the UK two-thirds of adults have a total cholesterol in excess of the recommended maximum of 5 mmol/L.

A developed country is one that is technologically advanced and whose population enjoy a relatively high standard of living. All countries in Europe are 'developed'.

Cholesterol is a major health issue across the world. In 2002, a report published by the World Health Organization (WHO) estimated that dyslipidaemia accounted for up to 8% of total diseases in developed countries. Worldwide, cholesterol causes around 4.4 million deaths each year (about 7.9% of the global total).

WHERE DOES THE UK STAND?

Although this graph is only looking at people with very high total cholesterol levels, it still shows that blood cholesterol levels in the UK are relatively high by international standards. In British adults aged 16 and over, the average total cholesterol is 5.5 mmol/L. In addition, as cholesterol levels tend to increase with age, older adults tend to have higher levels than younger adults. Not only are these levels higher than the recommended target of 5.0 mmol/L, they are also substantially higher than those of many other countries. In China for example, average cholesterol is only 4.5 mmol/L in people aged 35–64 years.

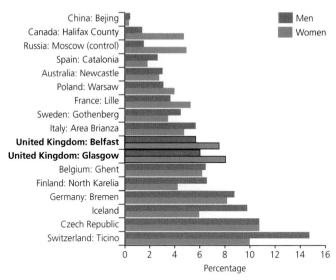

THE PERCENTAGE OF ADULTS AGED 35–64 WITH BLOOD CHOLESTEROL LEVELS GREATER THAN 7.8 MMOL/L (MONICA).

WHAT DOES HAVING HIGH CHOLESTEROL MEAN?

On the face of it, having raised cholesterol may not seem to be too alarming a prospect. Chances are, you will not even have any symptoms. You may be tempted to put your high cholesterol to the back of your mind and carry on regardless. This is the worst thing you can do. By ignoring the problem you are putting yourself at serious risk of developing cardiovascular disease. The WHO estimates that over 50% of cardiovascular disease in developed countries can be related to blood cholesterol levels in excess of 3.8 mmol/L (the theoretical minimum level).

In the UK, 66% of men and 67% of women have blood cholesterol levels in excess of 5.0 mmol/L.

*High cholesterol is **the** major risk factor for cardiovascular disease.*

Risk factors for cardiovascular disease include:

- having high LDL cholesterol and/or low HDL cholesterol and raised triglycerides
- advancing age
- having a history of cardiovascular disease in your family
- smoking
- being overweight
- having diabetes
- having high blood pressure
- being physically inactive.

CORONARY HEART DISEASE

In 2003, over 114,000 people died as a result of coronary heart disease in the UK alone. That's nearly 3.5 times more deaths than lung cancer.

Coronary heart disease (CHD) occurs when the arteries supplying blood to the heart become narrowed by atherosclerosis, causing angina and, sometimes a heart attack. It is the UK's biggest killer. Most deaths from CHD are because of a heart attack.

A staggering 2.7 million people are estimated to be living with CHD in the UK – a number that is rising year by year. This reflects our poor risk factor profile, our poor eating habits, our increasingly sedentary lifestyle or our plain complacency when it comes to dealing with our health. There is some good news however. Death rates from CHD have been falling in the UK since the late 1970s. Although more people than ever are living with CHD, less of us are dying from it. This is mainly because of improvements in the way in which we treat heart disease.

The INTERHEART study

One of the largest investigations into the worldwide incidence of coronary heart disease – the INTERHEART study – was published in 2004. INTERHEART gathered information from 52 different countries and included over 30,000 people. It was found that nearly 50% of heart attacks could be linked to abnormal levels of blood cholesterol. People with abnormal cholesterol levels were more than three-times more likely to have a heart attack than those with normal cholesterol levels.

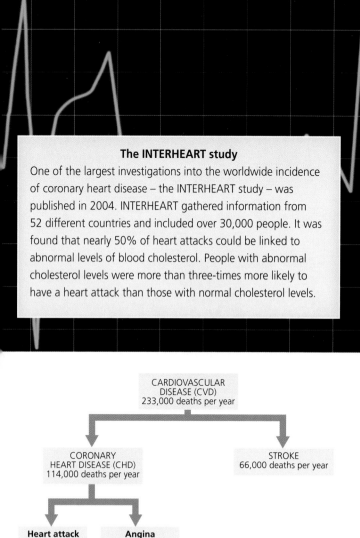

CARDIOVASCULAR
DISEASE (CVD)
233,000 deaths per year

CORONARY
HEART DISEASE (CHD)
114,000 deaths per year

STROKE
66,000 deaths per year

Heart attack
259,500 attacks
per year

Angina
341,500 new cases
per year

THE INCIDENCE OF CARDIOVASCULAR DISEASE IN THE UK.

THE NORTH/SOUTH DIVIDE

Within the UK, Scotland has the highest rate of CHD. The premature death rate for CHD for men living in Scotland is almost 67% higher than in the South West of England and around 84% higher for women. Scotland has held this unenviable position since the 1980s. The map below shows that the situation also tends to worsen the further north you travel.

So why is heart disease more common in northern Britain? The issue is a complicated

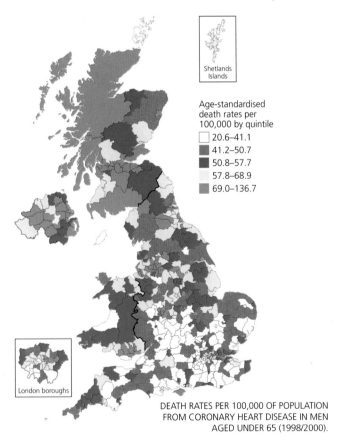

Shetlands Islands

Age-standardised death rates per 100,000 by quintile

- 20.6–41.1
- 41.2–50.7
- 50.8–57.7
- 57.8–68.9
- 69.0–136.7

London boroughs

DEATH RATES PER 100,000 OF POPULATION FROM CORONARY HEART DISEASE IN MEN AGED UNDER 65 (1998/2000).

one. The most obvious culprits are differences in eating habits and the popularity of meals which are high in fat, sugar and salt and low in fruit and vegetables. Smoking and binge-drinking habits may also contribute, although it is hoped that the impending ban on smoking in the workplace in Scotland may help many smokers to give up.

- Scottish people eat on average 153 grams of fruit and vegetables a day, compared with 198 grams a day in the South West of England.
- 35% of men and 28% of women in Scotland smoke, compared with 27% of men and 24% of women in England.
- 27% of women in Scotland drink more than the recommended daily maximum compared with 15% in London.
- 43% of Scottish men and 32% of Scottish women are overweight.

THE FRENCH PARADOX

Eating habits may go a long way to explain the high incidence of heart disease in countries like Scotland. Yet in France, where the enjoyment of fine foods is paramount, fewer people die from CHD than anywhere else in Europe. This is called the French paradox.

In France there are just 57 deaths per 100,000 people from CHD each year, compared with 188 per 100,000 in the UK.

Explaining the French paradox has baffled scientists for years and the answer remains largely unclear. Many experts believe that the apparent discrepancy could be in part due to the different attitudes to food and drink across the channel (although the way in which 'cause

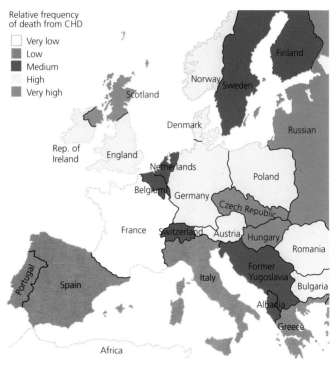

DEATH RATES FROM CORONARY HEART DISEASE ACROSS EUROPE.

In France, fat intake is similar to other European countries, but death from CHD is low. This is called the French paradox.

of death' is recorded on death certificates in France may also have something to do with it). Other experts argue that these days, eating habits in France are not so different to those in the UK, and the CHD death rate in France may be about to 'catch-up' with that in other countries.

In stark contrast to our eating habits in the UK, the French take time over their food. Rather than a hurried 're-fuelling', mealtimes are often the focal point of the day and can last for hours at a time. In France, people tend to prepare their food from scratch using fresh ingredients and 'ready-meals' are virtually unheard of.

People living in France, as well as those living in other countries like Italy, Spain and Greece, traditionally eat a 'Mediterranean diet'. This is a diet that is rich in monounsaturated fats (like olive oil), oily fish (like sardines, mackerel and salmon), vegetables and fruit. Some of these foods are a good source of omega-3 fatty acids which help to protect you against heart disease.

The French attitude to alcohol may also help to protect against heart disease. Drinking a moderate amount of alcohol on a regular basis (i.e. wine with meals) may help to raise levels of HDL cholesterol. Many experts believe that antioxidants found in red wine (as well as fruits and vegetables) can help to prevent the

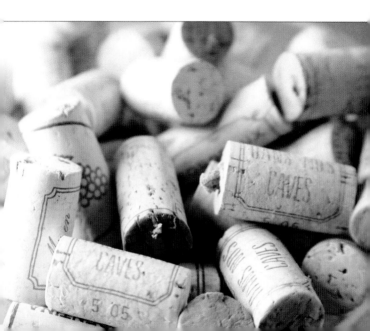

WHY THE FRENCH SHOULD BE AT MORE RISK OF CHD	WHY THE FRENCH MAY BE PROTECTED FROM CHD
• Consume rich, 'high-fat' foods like pastry, cheese, butter, cream and meat. • Smoking is as common as it is in the UK. • Blood pressure is as high as it is in the UK. • Drink alcohol to excess.	• Smaller portion size. • Different eating patterns. • Fresher ingredients prepared from scratch. • 'Mediterranean diet' with more. fruit and vegetables. • Drink alcohol on a regular basis. • Binge-drinking is uncommon.

build-up of fatty deposits in the arteries (atherosclerosis), but this is unproven. The popularity of 'binge-drinking' in the UK represents the flip side of the coin. The difference between French and British drinking habits is clearly illustrated by the changes in blood pressure over the course of the week. In the UK, blood pressure is usually higher on a Saturday, Sunday and Monday morning, after a weekend of overindulgence. In France, blood pressure remains at a constant level throughout the week.

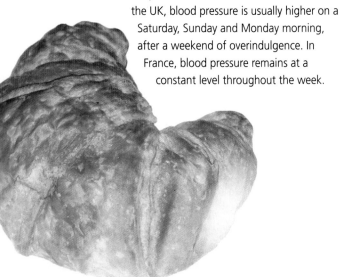

HOW DID I GET HIGH CHOLESTEROL?

There are a number of possible reasons why your cholesterol may be too high. The level of cholesterol in your bloodstream depends upon:

- age
- gender
- genetic factors
- having other illnesses like diabetes
- family history
- what you eat
- how active you are.

Whilst some of these factors are beyond your control, others are not. We may not be able to hold back the passage of time or alter our genetic make-up, but we can change what we eat and how much exercise we do. It is important to try to lower your cholesterol by whatever means you can.

AGE

Raised cholesterol is to some extent, a natural consequence of the ageing process. Or to look at it another way, the older you are, the more time you have had to do damage to your body! Raised cholesterol increases with age in both men and women. The graph overleaf shows the proportion of UK men and women with high cholesterol (greater than 5 mmol/L) split into age groups in 2003. Notice that the cholesterol levels peak in different age brackets for men and women. For men, the highest levels of cholesterol are observed between the ages of 45 and 54, whereas for women,

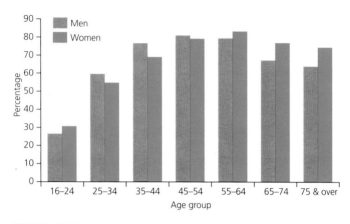

PERCENTAGE OF ADULTS WITH BLOOD CHOLESTEROL LEVELS OF 5.0 MMOL/L AND ABOVE (ENGLAND, 2003).

cholesterol is highest between the ages of 55 and 64. This trend is reflected in the rate of heart disease between the different sexes, with the onset of CHD in women tending to lag about 10 years behind that in men.

DIET

A sterol is a type of lipid, such as cholesterol, that is found in the cell membranes of plants and animals.

The people most at risk of having raised cholesterol are those who have a high amount of saturated fat in their diets. Saturated fats (found in foods such as meat, butter, cheese and cream) increase levels of LDL cholesterol in the bloodstream. However, eating healthily can reduce cholesterol levels by 5–10% and often considerably more. Reducing your intake of saturated fats (substituting these with poly- and monounsaturated fats) and eating more fruit, vegetables, salad, plant sterols and soya can all help. Healthier cooking techniques such as grilling rather than frying foods are also highly recommended. More advice on healthy eating can be found in the Managing Your Cholesterol Levels section. Remember that maintaining a healthy weight for your height (and crucially a healthy waist circumference) is also associated with other health benefits.

FAMILY HISTORY

Familial hypercholesterolaemia (FH) is the term used to describe one syndrome of high cholesterol that is inherited, passed from one generation to the next. In this instance, your high cholesterol is determined by a faulty gene and there is nothing you can do to avoid getting it (but of course, that's not to say that nothing can be done about it). FH is relatively

Familial hypercholesterolaemia is a disorder of high cholesterol that runs in your family.

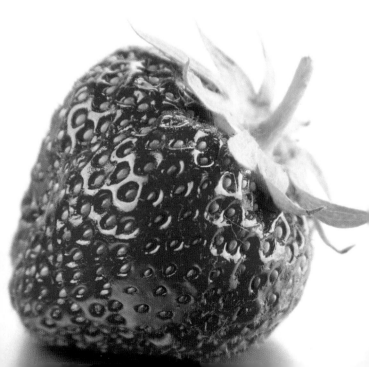

common in the UK and affects one person in every 500, that's approximately 120,000 people (nearly twice the capacity of a large Premiership Football Club stadium such as Old Trafford [Manchester United]).

People with FH have very high levels of cholesterol (usually 8–12 mmol/L, sometimes more and occasionally less!). The faulty gene means that their liver is unable to keep levels of LDL cholesterol as low as they should be which leaves people with FH more at risk of developing atherosclerosis and hence cardiovascular disease. FH starts at birth and persists throughout life.

FH is a very manageable condition that needs to be controlled with drug treatment and a healthy lifestyle. Clearly, it is vitally important to detect FH as early as possible so that appropriate treatment can be started and cardiovascular risk lowered. If one of your close relatives has recently been diagnosed with FH, you should have a cholesterol test. Other types of inherited lipid disorders include:

Screening programmes are under development to try and identify people with FH.

- familial hypertriglyceridaemia (excessively high levels of triglycerides)
- familial combined hyperlipidaemia (excessively high levels of cholesterol and triglycerides).

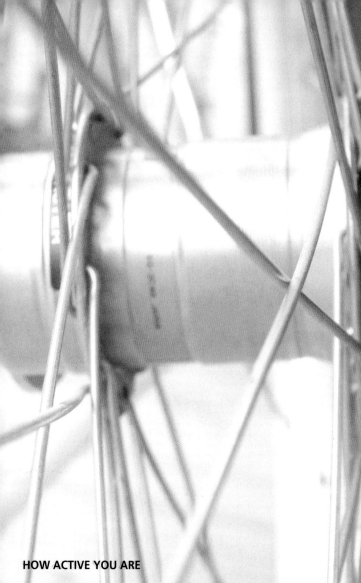

HOW ACTIVE YOU ARE

The health benefits associated with staying active are virtually limitless. Exercising regularly goes hand-in-hand with maintaining a healthy weight, which itself goes hand-in-hand with lowering your cardiovascular risk.

COMMON MISCONCEPTIONS ABOUT CHOLESTEROL

All cholesterol is bad for you.

This is not necessarily the case. We all need some cholesterol to help our bodies function properly. There's 'good' (HDL) cholesterol and 'bad' (LDL) cholesterol. LDL cholesterol is bad only when in excess. Saturated fats found in foods like meat, cheese, cream, butter and pastries tend to raise levels of LDL cholesterol in our bloodstream. In contrast, HDL cholesterol protects us against cardiovascular disease.

Slightly raised or normal cholesterol does not need our attention.

This is another myth. Patterns of low HDL cholesterol and raised triglycerides are often found in people with both normal and raised total cholesterol. In addition, whatever level of cholesterol you have, if you experience a cardiovascular event such as a heart attack, or stroke, your cholesterol should be lower.

High cholesterol only affects men.

This is most definitely not true. Women are just as likely to have high cholesterol as men, although perhaps at a slightly older age. The onset of cardiovascular disease (one of the causes of which is high cholesterol) in women tends to lag about 10 years behind that in men.

Using margarine instead of butter will help to lower your cholesterol.

Both margarine and butter are high in fat, so both should be used in moderation. Margarines made from unsaturated fats can help to lower cholesterol if eaten as part of a healthy diet. Margarine spreads like Benecol® and Flora Pro-Activ® that have been enriched with plant sterols and stanols can also help to lower cholesterol.

Thin people don't need to worry about their cholesterol.

Whilst people who are overweight are perhaps more likely to have high cholesterol or an abnormal lipid profile, people of a normal weight can also be at risk. Obesity is only one of a number of risk factors that can lead to cardiovascular disease.

People who need to lower their cholesterol should avoid eating eggs.

Whilst eggs are relatively high in cholesterol, dietary cholesterol has less impact on the level of cholesterol in your bloodstream than the saturated fat you eat. Eggs are a good source of protein, iron and vitamins A and D. Eating three or four eggs a week is fine as part of a healthy, balanced diet.

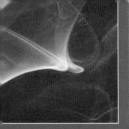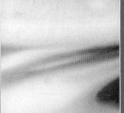

CHOLESTEROL MILESTONES

1755 The physician Albrecht von Haller discovers a soft yellow substance in the arteries of a corpse when conducting a post-mortem. He is the first to coin the term 'atheroma' (derived from 'athere' – the Greek for porridge-like mush or gruel).

1912 The American doctor, James Herrick establishes that blood clots in the coronary arteries can cause a heart attack by cutting off the heart's blood supply.

1930s An improved standard of living and increased cigarette smoking produce a sudden increase in the incidence of heart disease. The availability of fatty foods and meat all contribute to this upsurge.

1950s It is recognised that plant sterols lower the concentration of cholesterol in the blood.

1956 Dr Ancel Keys becomes the first person to establish a link between dietary fat and cholesterol.

1961 In the USA, the Framingham heart study establishes a link between cholesterol levels, blood pressure and an increased risk of heart disease.

1968 The drug cholestyramine is used to lower cholesterol levels in the blood.

1977 The effects of LDL and HDL cholesterol are first described, using data from the Framingham study.

1985 Joseph Goldstein and Michael Brown receive the Nobel Prize in Physiology for Medicine for their work on LDL cholesterol.

1990s Statins are introduced to lower cholesterol. These drugs have since revolutionised the prevention and treatment of cardiovascular disease.

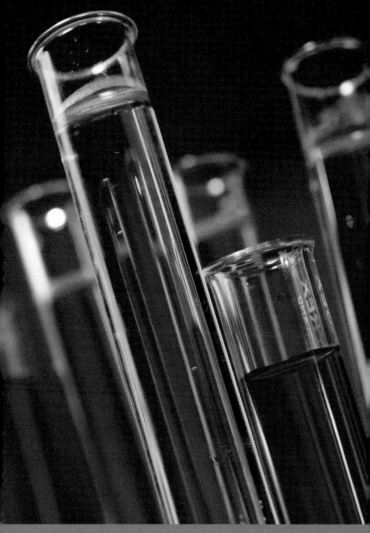

simple science

SIMPLE SCIENCE

If the levels of LDL cholesterol circulating in your bloodstream become too high, then excess cholesterol accumulates in the walls of your arteries.

Having excess LDL cholesterol in your bloodstream can increase your chances of developing cardiovascular disease. High cholesterol is sometimes referred to as a 'silent killer' because it quietly gets worse over many years without drawing our attention and the first we know of it is when we have a heart attack or other cardiovascular episode. But when does having high cholesterol actually start to threaten our lives? When the gradual build-up of cholesterol in the walls of our arteries (a process known as atherosclerosis) impedes the flow of blood we may suffer symptoms of angina, heart attack, stroke or peripheral arterial disease (PAD).

What is the difference between a heart attack and a stroke? Both occur as a result of the blockage of blood flow through an entire artery, but heart attacks and strokes affect different parts of the body.

- A heart attack occurs when the blockage is in the arteries (the coronary arteries) that supply the heart muscle with oxygen and blood.
- A stroke occurs when a blood clot blocks a blood vessel supplying part of the brain with oxygen and blood.

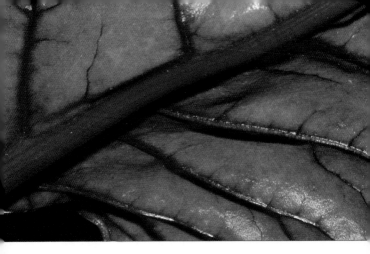

ATHEROSCLEROSIS

Atherosclerosis – the hardening or thickening of the arteries – is directly related to high levels of cholesterol in our bloodstream.

Atherosclerosis starts with the development of a plaque (atheroma), a fatty deposit that grows within the inner wall of an artery. These plaques build up over time and can gradually obstruct the flow of blood through the artery. Plaques can be fragile structures which can split or rupture attracting blood platelets (the tiny particles that help blood to clot properly) and this can lead to the formation of blood clots on the surface of the plaque, which further obstruct the artery and impede blood flow. The whole process can be broken down into a number of key stages (see overleaf).

'Atherosclerosis' comes from the Greek words 'athere' (meaning gruel or paste) and 'sklerosis' (meaning hardness).

49

THE KEY STAGES OF ATHEROSCLEROSIS

1 Cholesterol enters small breaks in the inner lining of the artery (called the endothelium).

2 Cholesterol and other substances become trapped in the damaged area.

3 LDL cholesterol is changed chemically (a process known as 'oxidation').

4 Monocytes (the largest type of white blood cell) are attracted to the site of injury.

5 Monocytes mature into macrophages (a large type of cell that 'gobbles up' unwanted particles).

6 Macrophages soak up the changed LDL cholesterol and are transformed into 'foam cells' inside the artery walls.

7 The foam cells die, releasing cholesterol which is seen as fatty deposits or 'streaks' inside the wall of the artery.

8 Muscle cells secrete fibrous tissue to try and wall-off the cholesterol deposits.

9 Over time the fatty streaks grow into plaques ('fibro fatty' structures) and start to restrict the flow of blood through the artery.

10 A plaque may split or rupture in time due to the mechanical forces acting on it from without, and the chemical processes operating on it from within.

11 Platelets in the blood are attracted to the site and start to make blood clot.

12 In the worst cases, this 'lesion' can completely cut off the flow of blood through the artery and cause a medical emergency.

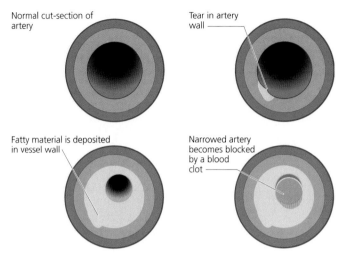

Normal cut-section of artery

Tear in artery wall

Fatty material is deposited in vessel wall

Narrowed artery becomes blocked by a blood clot

THE PROCESS OF ATHEROSCLEROSIS.

HOW DO CHOLESTEROL-LOWERING DRUGS WORK?

The term 'cholesterol lowering' is slightly misleading when it is used to describe the drugs that are used to treat cholesterol problems. Whilst these drugs do lower levels of LDL (and total) cholesterol, they do not necessarily lower levels of 'good' (HDL) cholesterol as well. In fact most drugs may actually increase HDL cholesterol. For the purposes of this book however, we will refer to cholesterol medications as 'cholesterol-lowering drugs'.

STATINS

The statin drugs (e.g. atorvastatin [Lipitor®] and simvastatin [Zocor®, Zocor Heart-Pro®]) work by blocking the manufacture of cholesterol in the liver. Statins are the most potent cholesterol-lowering drugs although they're less effective than the fibrates at reducing levels of triglycerides.

Cholesterol production is controlled by a number of biological catalysts called enzymes. The enzyme that controls the production of cholesterol is called hydroxymethylglutaryl coenzyme A (HMG-CoA) reductase, which is a bit of a mouthful and one of the reasons why these drugs are referred to simply as 'statins'! The statins work by preventing HMG-CoA reductase from working properly. This, in turn, means that less cholesterol is produced by the liver, and consequently, there is less cholesterol circulating in the bloodstream. The statins also appear to reduce the risk of heart disease by other mechanisms, in particular keeping the lining of blood vessels healthy.

Enzymes speed up specific biological reactions but are not themselves used up in the process.

FIBRATES

Although the fibrates (e.g. fenofibrate [Lipantil®]) have been around for many years, it is only recently that we have developed a better understanding of how they work. Fibrates exert their effects in the liver, where they block the production of triglycerides, and in the tissues of the body, where they increase the breakdown of triglycerides. Lowering levels of triglycerides also helps to raise levels of 'good' HDL cholesterol.

RESINS

Instead of targeting cholesterol itself, the resins (e.g. colestyramine [Questran®], colestipol [Colestid®]) attach themselves to bile acids.

Bile acids are made from cholesterol in the liver and are stored in the gall bladder (a small pear-shaped organ on the underside of the liver). Every time we eat a meal, bile acids are released from the gall bladder to help absorb any fat we have consumed. Under normal circumstances, 90–95% of these bile acids are recycled by the liver. However, by attracting the bile acids to them, resins help to remove them from the body in the faeces. If the body cannot reuse the old bile acids then it must make new ones. To do this, it needs more cholesterol, which it draws from the bloodstream into the liver, inadvertently reducing the amount of cholesterol in the blood. Resins are also known as anion exchange resins and bile acid sequestrants.

Bile is produced by the liver to help with the digestion of food in the gut.

SELECTIVE CHOLESTEROL ABSORPTION INHIBITORS

Ezetimibe (Ezetrol®) is in a new class of lipid-lowering drug, and acts by inhibiting the absorption of cholesterol in the intestines, or gut. It works on both dietary and biliary sources of cholesterol. If less cholesterol is absorbed from the food we eat, then less cholesterol finds its way to the liver. Because ezetimibe works in a completely different way to the statins, the two types of drugs are often given to patients at the same time in order to maximise the overall therapeutic effect.

NICOTINIC ACID

A form of vitamin B, nicotinic acid occurs naturally in a number of foods. By preventing the release of fatty acids from stores of fat within the body, nicotinic acid (Niaspan®) and closely-related substances like acipimox (Olbetam®) limit the amount of raw material the liver has available to it to make triglycerides. It also helps to lower LDL cholesterol and triglyceride levels whilst increasing levels of HDL cholesterol.

If you would like to learn more about the science surrounding cholesterol you can refer to BESTMEDICINE Lipid Disorders, available from www.bestmedicine.com

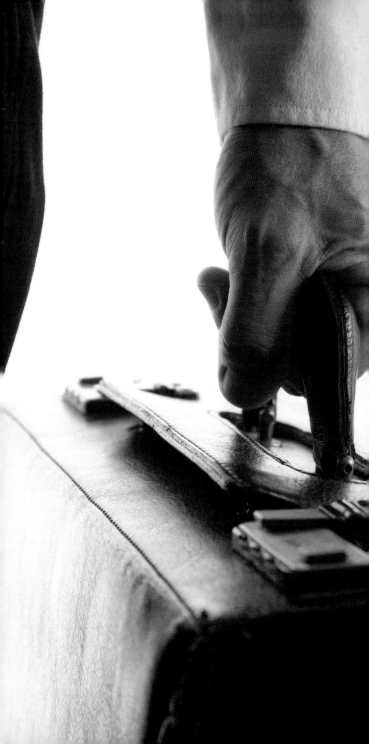

OMEGA-3 FISH OILS

Omacor® and Maxepa® are preparations of fatty acids that have been derived from omega-3 fish oils. Fish like kippers, mackerel, pilchards, sardines and salmon are rich in these oils. These substances mainly act in the liver to block the production of triglycerides.

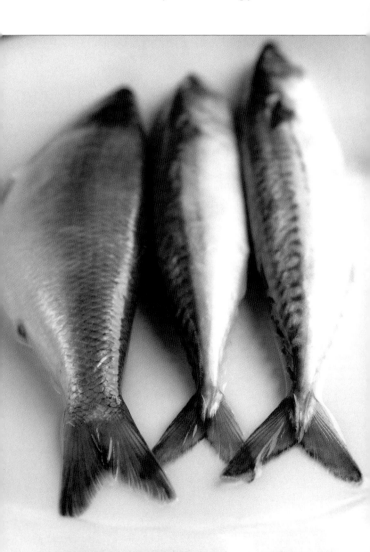

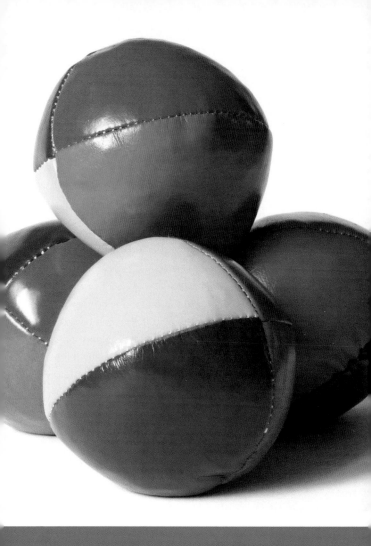

managing your cholesterol levels

MANAGING YOUR CHOLESTEROL LEVELS

Controlling your cholesterol levels so that they remain within recommended guidelines brings with it a number of important health benefits.

HOW WILL HAVING ABNORMAL CHOLESTEROL AFFECT MY LIFE?

If you manage your cholesterol effectively then it should not impact too heavily on your day-to-day way of living. Of course for many people this means taking care to manage something that as yet, has not caused them any health problems, or has even shown any symptoms. Finding the motivation to stick with your cholesterol-lowering programme can sometimes be difficult under these circumstances. Bear in mind however that there is no doubt that reducing the levels of 'bad' (LDL) cholesterol and triglycerides and raising levels of 'good' HDL cholesterol in your bloodstream will drastically reduce your risk of experiencing a heart attack or a stroke. There have been lots of long-term trials involving thousands and thousands of people that confirm that by controlling your cholesterol you not only significantly increase your chances of living longer but also help to ensure that the life you lead will be more disease-free.

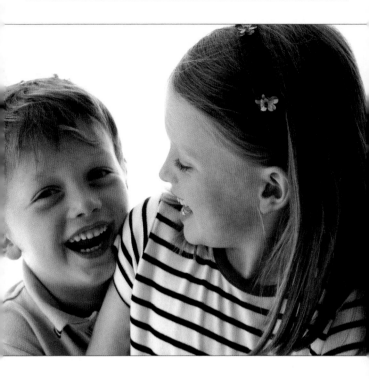

The lifestyle modifications that are required to manage cholesterol also benefit your general health in many other ways, like lowering your blood pressure and keeping you in shape. Feeling fitter in general should spur you on. Making lifestyle changes can be much easier if the whole family joins in, and everyone can benefit from eating less saturated fat.

Knowing your cholesterol level (along with other numbers such as your blood pressure, body mass index [BMI] and waist circumference) will help you to keep track of your risk of developing cardiovascular disease.

CALCULATE YOUR OWN BODY MASS INDEX (BMI)

It's very simple to work out your own BMI, to see whether your weight has put you at risk of abnormal cholesterol levels. Grab a tape measure, a set of bathroom scales and a calculator and follow these two steps.

- Measure your height in metres. Multiply this number by itself and write down the answer.
- Measure your weight in kilograms. Divide it by the number you wrote down in the first step. *The number you get is your BMI.*

For example: If your height is 1.80 metres, when you multiply this by itself you get 3.24. If your weight is 80 kilograms, divide 80 by 3.24 to give 24.7.

As a general rule, for adults aged over 20:

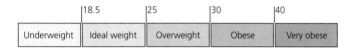

	18.5	25	30	40
Underweight	Ideal weight	Overweight	Obese	Very obese

Remember though that your BMI is only a broad indicator – it is affected by your body style – people with a very muscular build will have a higher BMI but may not be unhealthily fat. Your age and gender also affect your BMI. Some experts say that men can have a slightly higher BMI before they are at risk, probably due to the fact that they are usually more muscular than women. However, it is best to stick to the guidelines above – they are the internationally accepted boundaries for both genders. The BMI scale does not apply to children though, or during pregnancy.

MEASURING YOUR WAIST CIRCUMFERENCE

- The circumference (or distance around) your waist can provide a good indication of the amount of excess fat you have on your abdomen. Waist circumference is closely tied in with cardiovascular risk.
- Measure your waist circumference at the midpoint between the lower border of your ribs and the upper border of your pelvis.
- For men, a waist circumference greater than 102 cm (or 88 cm for women) indicates an increased health risk.

WHEN SHOULD I SEEK MEDICAL HELP?

High cholesterol does not usually have any noticeable symptoms. This can make it difficult to know whether or not to seek medical help in the first place. It is far more likely that high cholesterol will be picked up serendipitously during a routine health check. There are four main reasons why you may undergo a cholesterol test.

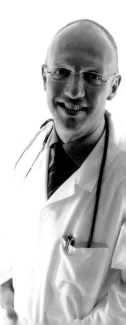

- You may be offered a cholesterol test as part of a general check on your health to assess your cardiovascular risk (opportunistic screening).
- You may be advised to have your cholesterol checked because you have other cardiovascular risk factors or have had a cardiovascular event.
- You display signs of dyslipidaemia (e.g. cholesterol deposits on eyelids or on tendons).
- You may have a relative who has recently been diagnosed with high cholesterol.

Only 28% of people aged 45–64 have had their blood cholesterol measured in the last 3 years.

Of course, you do not have to wait to be offered a cholesterol test. If you are concerned that your cholesterol may be abnormal, ask your doctor or practice nurse for a test.

SCREENING FOR FAMILIAL HYPERCHOLESTEROLAEMIA

Familial hypercholesterolaemia is an inherited cholesterol disorder that is passed from one generation to the next as a result of a faulty gene. Although nothing can be done to prevent it, if it is detected early enough with a simple blood test, then it can be managed with simple drug treatment.

The majority of people with familial hypercholesterolaemia are unaware that they have it.

Because high cholesterol does not often have any symptoms, people are often unaware that they have familial hypercholesterolaemia or indeed other inherited lipid disorders. They usually remain oblivious until they (or a family member), suffer a serious heart-related episode, usually at an earlier age than would otherwise be expected. Screening procedures are being evaluated to help rectify this shortfall and provide medical help to people who may not realise that they need it.

Diagnosing familial hypercholesterol-aemia can be difficult in children and sometimes a simple cholesterol test is not completely reliable. HEART UK recommends that children from affected families should be tested before the age of 10 but after the age of 2.

SIGNS OF FAMILIAL HYPERCHOLESTEROLAEMIA

- Cholesterol deposits on tendons (tendon xanthomata)
  - hard white deposits in tendons overlying knuckles
  - thickened Achilles tendons on back of ankles.
- Cholesterol deposits in skin around eye or on eyelid (xanthelasmata).
- Pale white ring around the rim of the iris of the eye (corneal arcus).

TESTING FOR CHOLESTEROL

The 'cholesterol test' is a simple blood test. From it, your doctor, practice nurse or pharmacist will be able to determine your **lipid profile**. This is:

- your total cholesterol
- your level of HDL cholesterol
- your level of triglycerides.

In most cases, the level of LDL cholesterol can be calculated from these values.

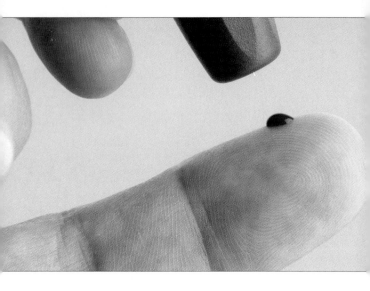

THE TEST PROCEDURE

When you visit your local surgery or pharmacy for a cholesterol test, it is likely that the person performing the test will follow a procedure similar to the one outlined on the next page. If you are having the full lipid profile measured, you will probably be told not to eat or drink anything (except water) for 12–14 hours before the test.

Your pharmacist may be able to measure your blood cholesterol levels.

Your GP or practice nurse will take a blood sample from your arm and send it to a laboratory for analysis. Desktop analysers that require only a pinprick of blood from your finger are sometimes used, and these can give immediate results. These devices provide less accurate results than those obtained from a laboratory.

THE CHOLESTEROL BLOOD TEST

1. You may be instructed not to eat for 12–14 hours before the test in order to accurately measure triglycerides as well as cholesterol.
2. You will be asked for a few personal details.
3. You will be asked to sit quietly for 10 minutes before you are tested.
4. Blood is taken from a vein on the inside of your elbow (or from your finger tip if using a desk top analyser).
5. Samples are sent away to a laboratory for processing (or if using a desktop analyser, the results will be known immediately).
6. You will be given a follow-up appointment (to discuss your results or to take a further measurement).
7. You will be offered advice whatever the outcome of your test.
8. Your doctor will discuss with you whether you are at risk of further complications, such as coronary heart disease.
9. You may be given a cholesterol management programme.

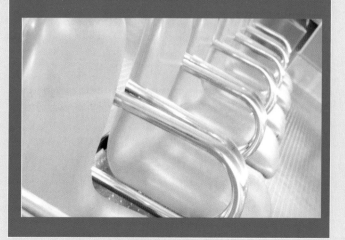

'IDEAL' cholesterol levels are currently described as total cholesterol of less than 5 mmol/L, with LDL cholesterol less than 3 mmol/L.

HOME TESTING KITS AND MOBILE SCREENING UNITS

Home testing cholesterol kits can falsely reassure you or make you unnecessarily anxious. Ideally, you should arrange a cholesterol test through your GP.

These days, kits for measuring cholesterol are widely available at pharmacies and even supermarkets. Whilst these kits can be a handy way of keeping track of your cholesterol, they are often not as accurate as the tests your doctor or practice nurse will be able to perform at your local surgery. If you take a home test, you will still have to go back to a healthcare professional, so that they can work out your risk of getting heart disease, and if appropriate, discuss the possibility of drug treatment with you.

HOME CHOLESTEROL TESTING/ MOBILE CHOLESTEROL SCREENING	
Pro's	Con's
Convenient	You will still need to go and see
Handy way of keeping track of	a doctor or nurse for further
your cholesterol.	advice.
	Not always accurate.
	You may (incorrectly) be given the 'all
	clear' and become complacent about
	your cholesterol.
	Do not offer follow-up appointments.

YOUR CHOLESTEROL MANAGEMENT PLAN

Once you have been diagnosed with high cholesterol, your doctor will work out the best way to lower your cholesterol and bring it back down to target levels, as defined by the Joint British Societies.

In general, there are two complementary management options.

1. Making lifestyle changes (which include following a cholesterol-lowering and healthy heart diet, increasing your levels of physical activity and stopping smoking).
2. Taking cholesterol-lowering drugs (as well as making the lifestyle changes listed above).

In order to work out which treatment approach is most suitable for you, your doctor will need to work out your cardiovascular risk.

The Joint British Societies publish national advice for health professionals and they include the British Cardiac Society, HEART UK, the British Hypertension Society, Diabetes UK and the Primary Care Cardiovascular Society.

New guidelines will soon set new target levels of total cholesterol less than 4 mmol/L and LDL cholesterol less than 2 mmol/L for those individuals whose cardiovascular risk is high.

67

CALCULATING YOUR CARDIOVASCULAR RISK

As mentioned previously, many factors determine how at risk you are of developing cardiovascular disease and the complications that are associated with it. High cholesterol is a very important contributing factor. A more extensive list includes:

- having raised LDL cholesterol, low HDL cholesterol, and/or raised triglycerides
- advancing age
- having a strong family history of cardiovascular disease
- smoking
- being overweight
- having diabetes
- having high blood pressure.

Your doctor may use a specialised chart like the ones here – developed by the Joint British Societies – to assess your cardiovascular risk over the next 10 years.

This chart should only be used to estimate cardiovascular risk in people who have not yet developed any symptoms of cardiovascular diseases such as angina, stroke or peripheral arterial disease (PAD). Because their cardiovascular risk is already high, people with diabetes need not be tested with the chart.

To estimate your risk, your doctor will:

1 Find the appropriate square that corresponds to your gender, age and smoking status.

CHARTS USED TO CALCULATE CARDIOVASCULAR RISK IN WOMEN.

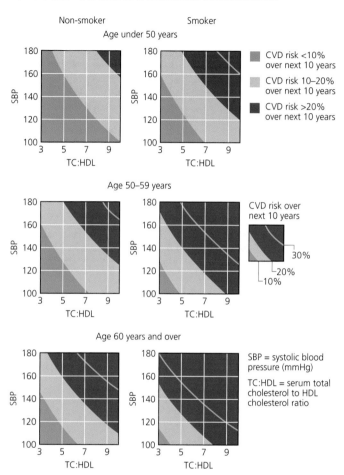

COURTESY OF THE UNIVERSITY OF MANCHESTER.

2 Determine where you lie within this square by plotting where your blood pressure and ratio of total cholesterol to HDL cholesterol (TC:HDL) meet.

3 Read off your 10-year cardiovascular risk.

CHARTS USED TO CALCULATE CARDIOVASCULAR RISK IN MEN.

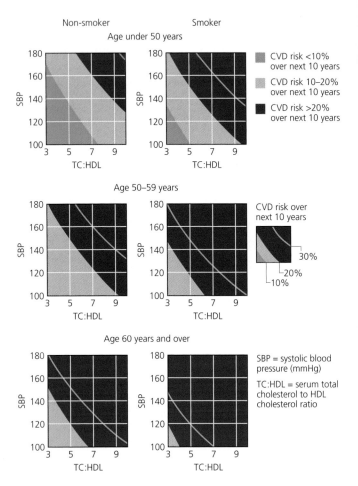

COURTESY OF THE UNIVERSITY OF MANCHESTER.

In order to be able to use these charts properly you need to calculate the ratio of your total cholesterol level to that of your HDL cholesterol. Your doctor or practice nurse will be able to help you with this.

WHAT DO THE COLOURS MEAN?

RED 10-year risk of cardiovascular disease exceeds 20%.

ORANGE 10-year risk is between 10 and 20%

GREEN 10-year risk is less than 10%

The traffic light bands determine whether you are at high (red), moderate (orange) or low (green) risk from cardiovascular disease within the next 10 years.

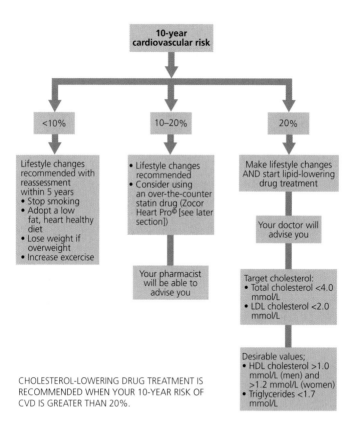

CHOLESTEROL-LOWERING DRUG TREATMENT IS RECOMMENDED WHEN YOUR 10-YEAR RISK OF CVD IS GREATER THAN 20%.

WILL I BE REFERRED?

Most people with cholesterol problems can be managed effectively in their local doctor's surgery. Rarely, it may be necessary to involve a specialist. This may apply to:

- people with extreme lipid values
- people who do not respond to conventional drug treatment
- people who cannot tolerate drug treatment
- people with familial hypercholesterolaemia or other inherited problems
- people who have high cholesterol for other reasons (e.g. liver or kidney disease, thyroid problems or diabetes).

TAKING CONTROL OF YOUR OWN CHOLESTEROL

Always remember that the most important member of your cholesterol management team is you.

- The more you learn about high cholesterol, the easier it will be to manage it. Reading this book is a good start!
- Take an active role in the management programme which your doctor devises for you – ask lots of questions.
- Act on the advice you are being offered.
- Be aware of the potential complications of high cholesterol, and look out for early warning signs.
- Always attend the check-up appointments you are given.

LIFESTYLE CHANGES

If you have been diagnosed with high cholesterol, one of the first things that your doctor or healthcare provider will ask you to do is to modify your lifestyle. However simple these lifestyle measures may sound, they could end up saving your life by preventing you from having a heart attack or other life-threatening episode. Cholesterol-friendly lifestyle changes may include:

- following a cholesterol-lowering and heart-healthy diet
- losing weight if you are overweight
- exercising regularly
- giving up smoking.

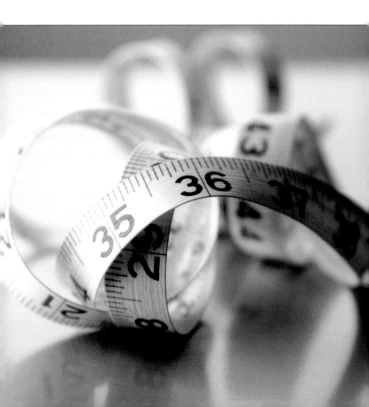

DIETARY ADVICE

The key to controlling your cholesterol lies in eating a balanced and healthy diet.
Replacing saturated fat (found in butter, cream, fatty meats and pastries) with mono- or polyunsaturated fats and oils is sensible. Of course, eating healthily will also help you to maintain a healthy weight for your height but you must watch the portion size. Tips for a cholesterol- and heart-friendly diet include eating:

- less fat (choosing low-fat foods)
- specifically, less saturated fat (substitute with mono- and polyunsaturated fats, including omega-3 fats)
- two portions of fish per week of which one should be oily
- more fruit, vegetables and salad
- fresh rather than processed foods
- less salt (no more than 6 g of salt per day)
- less sugary foods (less refined sugar)
- more fibre (in wholegrain starchy foods and beans, peas, lentils)
- more products that contain plant sterols and stanols (see later section)
- more soya protein.

For dietary advice to help lower your cholesterol please refer to Simple Extras.

BODY SHAPE

If your BMI indicates that you are overweight, you can get a better idea of your cardiovascular risk from looking at your body shape. Evidence suggests that it is very important where the fat is stored in your body. For example, your cardiovascular risk is higher if your fat is stored around your waist (making you 'apple-shaped') than if it is mostly on your thighs and hips (making you 'pear-shaped').

   Work out if you are an apple or a pear!
- Measure your waist and your hips in cm.
- Divide your waist measurement by your hip measurement.
- If the answer is greater than 1.0 (men) or 0.8 (women) you are 'apple-shaped'.

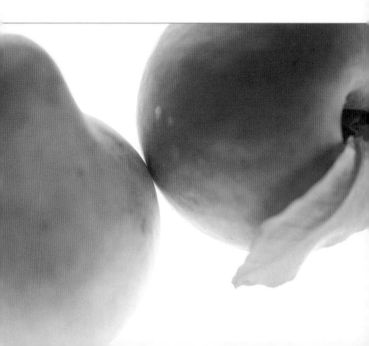

SALT CONTENT

Current advice suggests that you restrict your total salt intake to less than 6 grams per day (that's about 1 teaspoon). For most people this means cutting their daily salt intake in half.

Most processed foods, including breads and cereals, ready meals and sauces, contain large quantities of salt. This is why it's important to read food labels carefully and to be aware of how much hidden salt you are consuming. It's also another good reason to stick to freshly prepared foods wherever possible and avoid adding salt either when cooking or at the table.

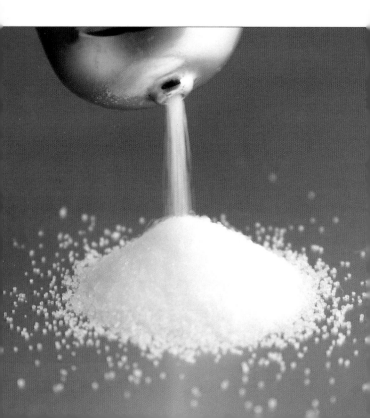

Type of fat	What do they do?	Where are they found?
UNSATURATED		
Monounsaturated	Help lower LDL cholesterol.	Rapeseed oil, olive oil, walnut oil, avocado, some margarines.
Polyunsaturated	Help lower LDL cholesterol.	Cornflower oil, sunflower oil, soya oil, some margarines.
Omega-3 (polyunsaturated fats) – marine sources	Help prevent potentially fatal heart rhythm changes. Help lower triglycerides and help prevent abnormal blood clotting.	Fish oil, oily fish (herrings mackerel, pilchards, sardines, salmon).
Omega-3 (polyunsaturated fats) – plant sources		Rapeseed oil, linseed oil, soya oil, walnuts, dark green vegetables.
SATURATED	Increase LDL cholesterol.	Butter, hard cheese, lard, dripping, suet, coconut oil, palm oil.

PLANT STEROLS AND STANOLS

Recently, we have been bombarded in the media with an ever-growing selection of so-called 'functional foods'. These include products like Benecol® and Flora Pro-Activ® – yoghurts, milk, margarine, savoury spreads and snack bars that have been enriched with plant sterols or stanols.

Sterols are found naturally in vegetable oils, nuts, grains, seeds and vegetables and have a similar chemical structure to cholesterol. Stanols are derived from tall tree oils. When eaten, these agents reduce the amount of cholesterol that the body can absorb, with the excess cholesterol passing out of the body untouched.

A sterol is a type of lipid, such as cholesterol, that is found in the cell membranes of plants and animals.

But do these products actually work? The evidence gathered to date suggests that they do. In an article published in the *British Medical Journal* in 2000, it was revealed that adding plant sterols or stanols to margarine reduced LDL cholesterol by an average of:

■ 0.54 mmol/L in people aged 50–59
■ 0.43 mmol/L in people aged 40–49
■ 0.33 mmol/L in people aged 30–39.

These reductions may reduce the risk of heart disease by about 25% (substantially more than the reduction achieved by simply reducing your intake of saturated fat). So the benefits are clear, but at what cost? It has been estimated that incorporating these foods into your diet will cost you an extra £70 a year, that's 20 pence per day, less than the cost of a newspaper.

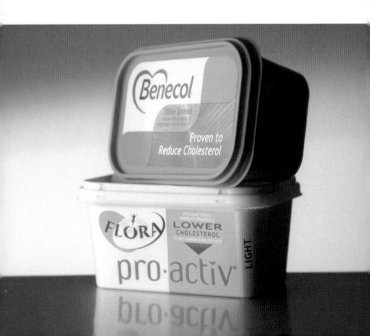

ALCOHOL

Research has shown that drinking alcohol in moderation can actually help to lower your risk of cardiovascular heart disease. Indeed, the health benefits associated with the odd glass of wine may help to explain why the French have such a good record when it comes to heart disease (see Why Me?). However, large amounts of alcohol can raise blood pressure and triglycerides and contribute to weight gain and other serious medical and social complications. Aim to drink alcohol in moderation (1–2 units daily and try some alcohol-free days).

Type of alcoholic drink (ABV [alcohol by volume])	How much?	How many units?
Average strength beer/lager	Half pint	1
Spirit	One pub measure (25 mL)	1
Wine (11–12% ABV)	Small glass (125 mL)	1.5
Beer/lager/cider – bottled	One bottle (330 mL)	1.5
'Alcopop' (4–6% ABV)	One bottle (330 mL)	1.3–2

EXERCISE

Use a pedometer to keep track of the number of steps you take each day.

As well as lowering your cardiovascular risk, lowering your weight and improving your general health, taking part in regular exercise can actually increase your levels of 'good' HDL cholesterol. Aerobic exercise, like brisk walking, jogging, cycling, swimming and dancing, is particularly good for people with high cholesterol. In contrast, anaerobic exercise like sprinting and weightlifting – in which the muscles use up oxygen faster than the blood can supply it – is not suitable for people at risk of heart disease.

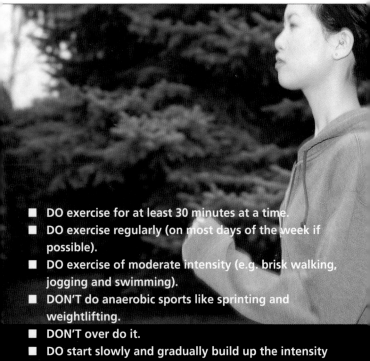

- **DO exercise for at least 30 minutes at a time.**
- **DO exercise regularly (on most days of the week if possible).**
- **DO exercise of moderate intensity (e.g. brisk walking, jogging and swimming).**
- **DON'T do anaerobic sports like sprinting and weightlifting.**
- **DON'T over do it.**
- **DO start slowly and gradually build up the intensity and duration of exercise.**
- **STOP immediately if you encounter chest pain or difficulty breathing.**

THE DRUG MANAGEMENT OF CHOLESTEROL

In addition to lifestyle changes, many people will also be prescribed cholesterol-lowering drugs to control their cholesterol and help prevent cardiovascular disease. Your doctor will usually recommend drug treatment if dietary changes by themselves have not improved your cholesterol as well as they would have hoped. If you are prescribed drug treatment, it is likely that you will have to remain on it for the rest of your life.

Your doctor will base any treatment decisions they make on national guidelines. If you have already developed diabetes, angina, had a heart attack or stroke, or have PAD, your doctor will want to prescribe you lipid-lowering medication. If you have not yet developed these conditions your doctor's decision will be based on your cardiovascular risk as assessed by charts like the one included earlier in this section. Whether or not you are prescribed cholesterol-lowering drugs depends on your risk of cardiovascular disease, not just your total, LDL and HDL cholesterol.

Drug treatment goes hand-in-hand with lifestyle changes and one should not replace the other.

The higher your cardiovascular risk, the more likely it is that your doctor will prescribe cholesterol-lowering drugs.

Those at highest risk are:

- people who have already been diagnosed with angina or who have had a heart attack
- people who have had bypass surgery or angioplasty
- people who have had a stroke
- people with PAD
- people with diabetes.

In the absence of these conditions, your cardiovascular risk is calculated from your total and HDL cholesterol and whether or not you:

- smoke
- have high blood pressure
- are of a certain age/gender
- have a family history of cardiovascular disease.
- are of a certain ethnic origin.

Sometimes, very high cholesterol is an isolated risk factor and is treated by itself (e.g. familial hypercholesterolaemia). In addition, there are other situations (e.g. kidney disease) where cholesterol-lowering drugs are recommended, and other complex situations in which people may require special treatment (e.g. people with HIV).

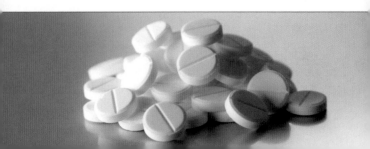

SO WHICH DRUGS WILL I BE PRESCRIBED?

Your doctor will take many factors into account in choosing which drug, or drugs, you will be treated with. Ultimately though, they will choose the type of drug that suits you the best. Drugs are grouped into a single class if they act in the same way. There are a wide range of cholesterol drugs currently available to treat people with cholesterol problems. These include:

Cholesterol-lowering drugs now cost the NHS more than any other type of drug.

- ■ statins (e.g. atorvastatin [Lipitor®] and simvastatin [Zocor®, Zocor Heart-Pro®])
- ■ fibrates (e.g. fenofibrate [Lipantil®] and gemfibrozil [Lopid®])
- ■ resins (e.g. colestyramine [Questran®], colestipol [Colestid®])
- ■ selective cholesterol absorption inhibitors (e.g. ezetimibe [Ezetrol®])
- ■ nicotinic acid (e.g. Niaspan®, Olbetam®)
- ■ omega-3 fish oils (e.g. Omacor®, Maxepa®)
- ■ combined treatments (e.g. simvastatin *plus* ezetimibe [Inegy®])

In general, statins are the first choice for treating hypercholesterolaemia (raised LDL cholesterol in the blood) and fibrates are first choice for treating hypertriglyceridaemia (raised triglycerides in the blood).

Whilst undergoing drug treatment, it is important that you have blood tests every 6–12 months to make sure that your cholesterol levels are being controlled by the drugs.

In 2004, the cost of prescriptions for cholesterol-lowering drugs was £769 million, an increase of £54 million since 2003.

Statins and fibrates are occasionally given together. This can be particularly helpful for treating people with mixed hyperlipidaemia, who have raised levels of both LDL cholesterol and triglycerides, in their blood. People taking statins and fibrates together will be monitored more often because the risk of side-effects is slightly greater.

Inegy® is a relatively new all-in-one product that combines both simvastatin and ezetimibe in the same tablet.

OTHER TYPES OF DRUG THAT CAN LOWER CARDIOVASCULAR RISK

If you have other conditions that are likely to increase your cardiovascular risk – like high blood pressure or type 2 diabetes – your doctor will probably recommend that you take drugs to treat them, if you are not doing so already. Blood pressure-lowering drugs include the beta-blockers (e.g. atenolol, bisoprolol) and the ACE inhibitors (e.g. enalapril, perindopril, ramipril).

If you would like to learn more about the drugs used to treat high blood pressure or type 2 diabetes, you can refer to A Simple Guide to Blood Pressure *and* A Simple Guide to Type 2 Diabetes.

STATINS

The statins (e.g. atorvastatin [Lipitor®], fluvastatin [Lescol®], pravastatin [Lipostat®], rosuvastatin [Crestor®], simvastatin [Zocor®]) are the most frequently prescribed drugs for the treatment of high cholesterol. Currently, around 1.8 million people in the UK take statins and it is estimated that these drugs save between 6,000 and 7,000 lives a year by preventing coronary complications alone.

You will normally be advised to take your statin at night. This is because the body produces most of its cholesterol whilst we are asleep (and are unable to obtain cholesterol from food yourself). Atorvastatin [Lipitor®] and rosuvastatin [Crestor®] can be taken at any time of the day.

Statins and the prevention of heart disease

A number of large clinical trials in which thousands of patients were treated with statins for a number of years, have shown that they can help to limit the number of people who die from cardiovascular disease, by reducing heart attacks and strokes. This has meant that statins are now recommended for all people with established cardiovascular disease and people who are at high risk of developing cardiovascular disease (especially smokers, and those people with diabetes, high blood pressure or a family history of premature death from heart disease).

Statins are recommended for people at high risk of cardiovascular disease.

FIBRATES

The fibrates (e.g. bezafibrate [Bezalip®], ciprofibrate [Modalim®], fenofibrate [Lipantil®] and gemfibrozil [Lopid®]) are used most often to treat people with raised levels of triglycerides and low levels of HDL cholesterol in their bloodstream. Fibrates can also be given together with statins to treat people with mixed hyperlipidaemia (raised LDL cholesterol and triglycerides). It is not recommended that people with liver or kidney disease take fibrates to control their cholesterol. Certain types of blood-thinning drugs may also react badly with fibrates. Your doctor will be able to advise you whether fibrates are the most suitable medication for you.

RESINS

The resins (e.g. cholestyramine (Questran®) and colestipol (Colestid®) are used to treat people with high levels of LDL cholesterol. Unlike the other cholesterol-lowering drugs, the resins are in the form of powders, which must be shaken vigorously with liquid in order to dissolve. These 'drinks' do not taste particularly pleasant and this may put a lot of people off taking the drugs. Flavouring the water using fruit juices may help to disguise the taste. As well as affecting the absorption of cholesterol within the body, resins may also interfere with the absorption of a number of important vitamins (e.g.

vitamin A, D and K). For this reason, people who take resins over long periods of time may be advised to take vitamin supplements.

Unlike the statins, resins can be used in children with elevated cholesterol. However, they are not recommended in people who have raised levels of triglycerides because they may aggravate the problem.

SELECTIVE CHOLESTEROL ABSORPTION INHIBITORS

A relatively new type of drug, ezetimibe (Ezetrol®), can be used to lower cholesterol in people who cannot take statins, or can be used as an additional drug for people who already take statins or fibrates. This is because ezetimibe works in a different way to statins or fibrates and adds to the cholesterol-lowering effect. Inegy® is a ready-made combination of ezetimibe and simvastatin and saves you having to take both drugs separately. The advent of ezetimibe has meant that fewer prescriptions for resins are now issued.

If you would like to learn more about the drugs used to treat cholesterol disorders you can refer to BESTMEDICINE Lipid Disorders, *available from www.bestmedicine.com*

THE SIDE-EFFECTS OF DRUG TREATMENT

The side-effects most often associated with the different classes of cholesterol-lowering drugs are summarised in the table overleaf. Generally speaking, cholesterol drugs are remarkably free from serious side-effects and most people can take them without experiencing any complications.

MUSCLE DAMAGE

Rarely, people who take statins or fibrates to lower their cholesterol report pain in their muscles. In a very few cases, this can lead to a serious disease called rhabdomylosis, in which the muscles themselves become badly damaged. Whilst rhabdomylosis is a potentially fatal condition – it is extremely rare. If you do experience severe muscular aches and pains whilst taking statins or fibrates, you should stop taking the drug immediately and consult your doctor. Usually the pains are generalised and similar to the aches and pains suffered during the first few days of flu.

If you are taking a combination of a statin and a fibrate to lower your cholesterol (or you are taking a very high dose of either drug), your risk of experiencing adverse muscle effects may be higher than normal.

LIVER DAMAGE

Very rarely people taking statins experience liver problems. For this reason your liver function should be tested before you embark on drug treatment and may be monitored at regular intervals afterwards. This is to make sure that the drug is safe to take and does not affect your liver. It is not recommended that people who drink a lot of alcohol take statins because they are already putting a lot of extra strain on their liver by drinking in the first place.

Liver functions tests are very straightforward. A blood sample is taken to determine whether the amount of an enzyme in the liver (called transaminase) has gone up – a sign that the liver may not be working properly. If the level rises too high then your doctor may take you off your statin.

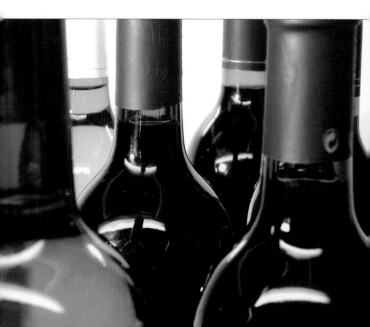

THE SIDE-EFFECTS MOST FREQUENTLY ASSOCIATED WITH CHOLESTEROL-LOWERING DRUGS

Drug type	Possible side-effects
Statins	Minor gastrointestinal disturbances. Rarely, muscular aches and pains (myalgia), muscle inflammation (myopathy or myositis) and very rarely muscle breakdown (rhabdomylosis) can occur. Rarely liver damage can occur.
Fibrates	Minor gastrointestinal disturbances. Rarely, muscle problems and very rarely rhabdomylosis have been reported.
Resins	Constipation, diarrhoea, nausea, and gastrointestinal discomfort.
Selective cholesterol absorption inhibitors	Rarely, minor gastrointestinal disturbances, rash, pancreatitis, allergic skin swelling.
Nicotinic acid	Diarrhoea, nausea, vomiting, abdominal pain, flushing, rash, liver abnormalities, worsening diabetes control.
Omega-3-fish oils	Minor gastrointestinal disturbances.

No drug treatment is without its side-effects. People may respond in slightly different ways to the same medicine. If you experience symptoms which you think may be due to the medication you are taking, you should talk to your doctor, pharmacist or nurse. If the side-effect is unusual or severe, your GP may decide to report it to the MHRA. The MHRA operates a 'Yellow Card Scheme' which is designed to flag up potentially dangerous drug effects and thereby protect your safety. The procedure has changed recently to allow patients to report adverse drug reactions themselves. Visit www.yellowcard.gov.uk for more information.

OBTAINING CHOLESTEROL-LOWERING DRUGS WITHOUT A PRESCRIPTION

In 2004, a low dose of simvastatin (Zocor Heart-Pro®) was made directly available to people at pharmacies without the need for a doctors prescription. The decision to supply simvastatin over-the-counter (OTC) took many people by surprise because it was fast-tracked with Government approval. There are a number of possible reasons for this.

In people at risk of CVD, the long-term use of even a low dose of simvastatin may reduce the risk of a coronary event by 10% after 1 year and by 33% after 3 years.

1. There is little doubt that reducing your cholesterol levels lowers the risk of cardiovascular disease and the evidence that the statins reduce cholesterol levels is irrefutable.
2. At its lowest available dose of 10 mg, simvastatin is not usually associated with any serious side-effects.
3. Supplying everybody who has cholesterol above recommended levels with a statin on prescription would place an enormous burden on NHS resources. This may have influenced the government's decision to make the drug available for people to buy.

Remember that buying a drug yourself is often more expensive than getting it with a prescription (especially if you don't usually pay for your prescriptions!). It is important to weigh up the extra cost against the benefits you will gain from taking Zocor Heart-Pro®. These will be different for everybody.

Over-the-counter (OTC) drugs can be obtained without a prescription from your pharmacist.

Preventative treatment

Lowering cholesterol by taking any statin on a regular basis may lower your risk of cardiovascular disease. Whilst the benefits of the sort of cholesterol-lowering that statins produce are clear, it is important that 'at-risk' people do not become complacent just because they are taking a drug treatment. It is still very important that you take preventative lifestyle measures too, like eating healthily, taking regular exercise and giving up smoking.

Your pharmacist can help you

Zocor Heart-Pro® is only available from pharmacies, and the pharmacist is required to ensure that you meet the criteria laid down by the authorities to ensure that the drug is appropriate for you. Your pharmacist will determine your risk of heart disease, by asking you a number of questions and may recommend that you have your weight, cholesterol and blood pressure measured too, before offering you the opportunity to buy Zocor Heart-Pro® (which you will probably need to take for the rest of your life, so you need to consider the long-term costs involved). If the outcome of your assessment is that you may be at a higher than moderate risk of heart disease, then Zocor Heart-Pro® may not be suitable for you and you will be referred to your GP.

If you decide to start taking Zocor Heart-Pro®, you should inform your GP when you next see him or her because all drugs have the potential to cause side-effects. As with all medicines, it is important that you take Zocor Heart-Pro® in accordance with its dosing instructions. Always read the information leaflet provided and make sure that you know what side-effects to look out for.

How safe is it?

Simvastatin has been available as a prescription only medicine (POM) since the late 1980s and many millions of people have been treated safely. As with all statins, there is a slight risk of severe muscle damage associated with simvastatin treatment. This is very rare and is more likely to occur at higher doses or when simvastatin is taken together with other cholesterol-lowering drugs. The dose of simvastatin in Zocor Heart-Pro® is the lowest available. However, if you experience any muscular aches and pains, it is important that you stop taking Zocor Heart-Pro® immediately and consult your doctor. Since your chances of developing muscle problems may be slightly increased if you consume a lot of grapefruit juice whilst taking simvastatin, this drink is best avoided.

THE DRUG DEVELOPMENT PROCESS

Developing and launching a new drug onto the commercial market is an extremely costly and time-consuming venture. The process can take a pharmaceutical company between 10 and 15 years from the outset, at an estimated cost of £500 million. Much of this time is spent fulfilling strict guidelines set out by regulatory authorities in order to ensure the safety and quality of the end product. Once registered, a new drug is protected by a patent for 20 years, after which time other rival companies are free to manufacture and market identical drugs, called generics. Thus, the pharmaceutical company has a finite period of time before patent expiry to recoup the costs of drug development and return a profit to their shareholders.

During the development process, a drug undergoes five distinct phases of rigorous testing – the preclinical phase, which takes place in the laboratory – and phases 1, 2, 3 and 4, which involve testing in humans. Approval from the regulatory body and hence, a licence to sell the drug, is dependent on the satisfactory completion of all phases of testing. In the UK, the Medicines and Healthcare Products Regulatory Agency (MHRA) and the European Medicines Evaluation Agency (EMEA) regulate the drug development process.

- Only about 1 in every 100 drugs that enter the preclinical stage progress into human testing because they failed to work or have unacceptable side-effects.
- Animal testing is an important part of drug development. Before a drug reaches a human, it is vital that its basic safety has been established in an animal. Researchers do everything in their powers to minimise the number of animals they use and must adhere to strict guidelines issued by the Home Office.
- Phase 1 testing takes place in groups of 10–80 healthy volunteers.
- Phase 2 testing takes place in 100–300 patients diagnosed with the disease the drug is designed to treat.
- Phase 3 clinical trials involve between 1,000 and 3,000 patients with the relevant disease, and look at both the short- and long-term effects of the drug.
- Phase 4 testing and monitoring continues after the drug has reached the market.

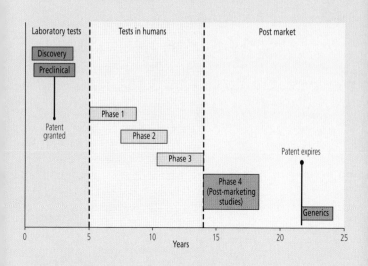

Laboratory tests	Tests in humans	Post market

Discovery

Preclinical

Patent granted

Phase 1

Phase 2

Phase 3

Phase 4
(Post-marketing
studies)

Patent expires

Generics

0   5   10   15   20   25
Years

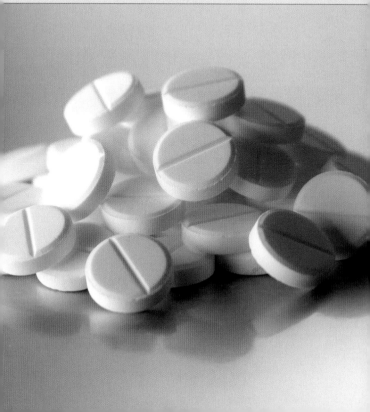

SPECIAL TREATMENT GROUPS

People with established cardiovascular disease

Even if you have previously experienced a heart attack or a stroke, it's not too late for lowering your cholesterol to make a difference to your health. In fact, it's even more important and may prevent you from having a further episode. If you have been diagnosed with coronary heart disease, as a matter of course you may be given:

- statins
- a daily dose of aspirin or clopidogrel (Plavix®) (both drugs make your blood less likely to form clots)
- blood pressure-lowering or antianginal drugs.

People with diabetes

Cardiovascular disease is easily the most common cause of death amongst people with diabetes. Because people with diabetes are already at a higher risk of cardiovascular disease than people without diabetes, they may automatically receive a cholesterol-lowering treatment.

People with FH and other inherited lipid disorders

People who have inherited lipid abnormalities will be treated slightly differently to the rest of the general population. Their treatment is usually more 'aggressive', which means that the following

are all the more important:
- ■ dietary changes (more intensive)
- ■ giving up smoking and exercising more
- ■ intensive drug treatment
- ■ close monitoring and regular check-ups.

Usually (unless they are pregnant or a child), people with familial hypercholesterolaemia will be given a statin straight away. Combination therapy with ezetimibe, fibrates or resins is also often used to magnify the cholesterol-lowering effect.

Instead of a statin, children with familial hypercholesterolaemia may be given a resin or ezetimibe in the first instance. Many children are switched to statins after they have passed puberty. Rather than drug treatment, young children can have their cholesterol controlled by being fed a low-fat diet, with lean meats, low-fat dairy products, fish, nuts, cereals, fruit and vegetables. A dietitian will be able to advise you how to strike the right balance.

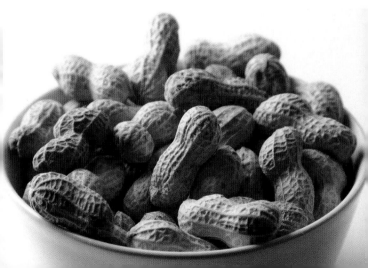

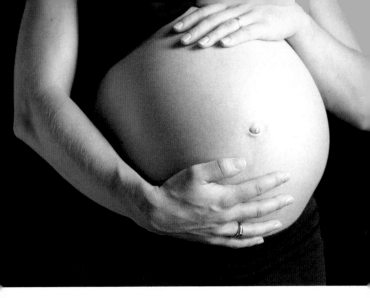

Women

Heart disease if often portrayed as a man's disease but women are just as likely to be affected, albeit at perhaps a slightly later stage in their lives. The slower onset of CHD in women may be related to the beneficial effects of the oestrogen hormone on heart health. Oestrogen may increase levels of HDL cholesterol and thereby offer some form of protection to women who have not yet undergone the menopause.

If your risk of cardiovascular disease is relatively high (for example because you have high cholesterol, you smoke, you have high blood pressure or heart disease runs in your family), your doctor may recommend that you do not take the combined oral contraceptive pill and instead consider alternative forms of contraception. This is simply a precaution because some clinical studies have identified a link between the contraceptive pill and heart disease.

Cholesterol-lowering drugs are not usually recommended during pregnancy. If you are pregnant, or are thinking about becoming pregnant, you should consult your doctor for further advice.

People with HIV

Some of the drugs used to treat people with HIV can cause cholesterol problems themselves. Taking these drugs (called antiretrovirals) for long periods of time can cause changes in body fat called 'fat redistribution', also known as 'lipodystrophy syndrome'. There are three general patterns of fat redistribution that are seen in people with HIV:

- **lipodystrophy** – gaining fat on the abdomen, shoulder blades or around the neck or in the breasts
- **lipoatrophy** – losing fat from under the skin which becomes obvious in the face, arms, legs and buttocks
- a mixture of both fat gain and fat loss.

People with HIV may be referred to an expert in treating dyslipidaemia.

These fat changes can be accompanied by metabolic changes (increases in the levels of cholesterol, fats and sugar in the blood).

Before prescribing you the antiretrovirals, your doctor will take into account your cholesterol levels and any other cardiovascular risk factors you may have.

SPECIAL TREATMENT GROUP	RECOMMENDATIONS
People with established cardiovascular risk	• Lowering your cholesterol can still make a difference, even if you have already had a heart attack.
People with diabetes	• Cardiovascular risk is high in the first place. • People with diabetes are more likely to be given cholesterol-lowering drugs.
People with familial hypercholesterolaemia	• Cholesterol-lowering is usually more 'aggressive'. • Statins are the drug of choice. • Children require slightly different management to adults.
Women	• Heart disease affects women as well as men. • If your cardiovascular risk is high, you may be advised not to take the contraceptive pill. • Cholesterol-lowering drugs are not usually recommended during pregnancy.
People with high blood pressure	• High blood pressure is also an important risk factor for CVD. • Blood pressure-lowering drugs can be taken at the same time as cholesterol-lowering drugs.
Elderly people (the over 70s)	• The prevention of CVD is important, no matter what your age. • Lipid-lowering drugs are just as useful in the elderly as they are in the general population.
People with HIV	• May be necessary to switch combination of antiretrovirals to avoid 'fat redistribution' and lipodystrophy syndrome. • Blood cholesterol levels should be monitored throughout treatment.
People with kidney disease	• Statins can be used but people who are on immunosuppressive drugs following a kidney transplant will need extra monitoring. • Fibrates not suitable.

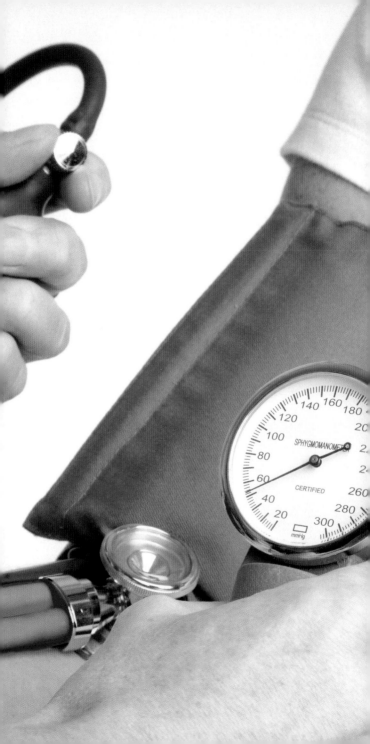

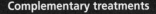

Complementary treatments

Complementary, or alternative, treatments can play an important part in the long-term management of high cholesterol. However, they should never replace the conventional cholesterol-lowering medications prescribed for you by your doctor. You should always keep your cholesterol management team informed of any alternative medication you are using to control your cholesterol, in case these interfere with the programme of care they are recommending.

The main reason that they are not recommended as 'stand-alone' methods of controlling cholesterol, is that the clinical evidence to back them up is often lacking. Claims regarding their effectiveness and safety are generally not reinforced by well-designed clinical trials performed in lots of people. This is in stark contrast to cholesterol-lowering drugs, which have to go through strict testing procedures before they can be widely used in people.

If you are considering using herbal supplements to control your cholesterol, always consider the advice of the Medicines Control Agency:

- never buy herbal products abroad or by mail order
- only buy a herbal remedy if it states clearly which herbs it contains
- stop using herbal remedies if you experience any side-effects
- do not exceed the stated dose
- do not use if you are pregnant or breast feeding.

COMPLEMENTARY THERAPIES THAT HAVE BEEN PROMOTED AS LOWERING CHOLESTEROL

Garlic	May help to reduce cholesterol and triglycerides.
Chromium/Brewer's yeast	May lower cholesterol.
Psyllium seed	
Fruit pectin	
Glucomannan	Sources of soluble fibre.
Beta-glucan (found in oat bran)	
Alpha-linolenic acid (ALA)	Source of omega-3 fatty acids.
Coenzyme Q-10	May help to relieve the muscle pain (myalgia) sometimes caused by cholesterol-lowering drugs.

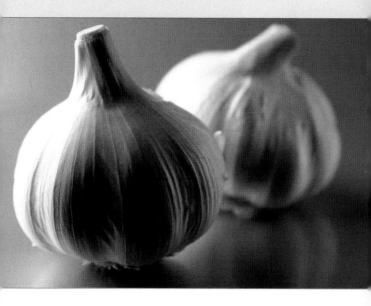

THE LONG AND THE SHORT OF IT

What should I expect?

Although abnormal lipids are strongly linked to cardiovascular heart disease, having an unhealthy lipid profile is by no means a death sentence. You can take steps to make sure it is controlled and does not become life-threatening.

Rather than a problem, try and see discovering that you have a lipid or cholesterol abnormality as an early warning sign and one that you are fortunate enough to have been made aware of. Remember that many people are unaware their cholesterol is too high before it becomes too late.

Although heart disease remains the UK's biggest killer, fewer people die from it these days than used to be the case. This is probably because of better awareness, better treatments and more effective management approaches.

Know your numbers

Most importantly, do not ignore your cholesterol level. By doing so you may be placing yourself at unnecessary risk. Instead, see controlling your cholesterol as an opportunity to take control of your health and well-being.

Know your other cardiovascular risk factors

Cholesterol is just one of a number of factors that can contribute to your chances of developing cardiovascular disease. As well as controlling your cholesterol, bear in mind the influence that your blood pressure, your weight, your diet and your lifestyle can have on your heart and circulation. It is important to be aware of and to tackle these factors together.

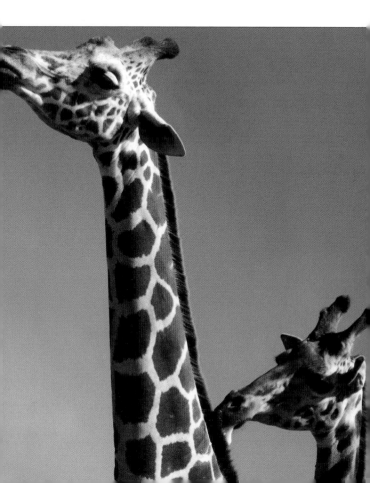

GETTING THE MOST OUT OF YOUR HEALTH SERVICE

Having abnormal lipids is a long-term condition that should be treated on a case-by-case basis. Maintaining a good relationship with your GP, or any other member of your cholesterol management team, is fundamental to managing your cholesterol effectively. These people will be able to explain to you why you have high cholesterol, teach you how best to manage it and help you protect yourself against cardiovascular disease.

It is important that you remain in regular contact with a member of your cholesterol management team. Remember, if one management approach fails to work, there are many others that can be tried.

HOW YOU CAN HELP YOUR NHS TO HELP YOU.

- Take your cholesterol level seriously.
- Take advantage of cholesterol checks when they are offered.
- Keep track of your cholesterol and arrange regular check-up appointments.
- Consider counselling if you or your family have a hereditary lipid disorder.

- If you are taking statins: Report any significant side-effects especially severe muscular aches and pains.

Visiting your doctor or any health care professional can sometimes be a confusing or daunting prospect. You may find that the consultation flies by and when your doctor asks if you have any questions, your mind goes blank. Writing down a list of questions before the consultation, or using the checklist below, may help you to get the most out of your appointment.

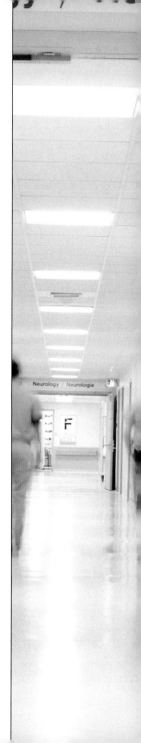

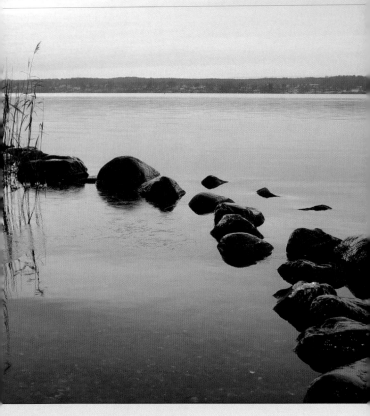

QUESTIONS TO ASK YOUR DOCTOR

- How high is my cholesterol?
- Am I at risk of developing heart disease?
- How can I lower my risk factors?
- Do I need to lose weight?
- Do I need to take medication?
- What's the best treatment for me? Are there any side-effects?
- By how much will this drug lower my cholesterol?
- What will happen if this treatment doesn't work?
- What are the side-effects of treatment?
- Which types of food should I be eating?
- Will my family have high cholesterol just because I have it?
- Did I inherit high cholesterol myself?
- Will lowering my cholesterol make me feel any different?
- If I already have heart disease, is there any point to me trying to lower my cholesterol?

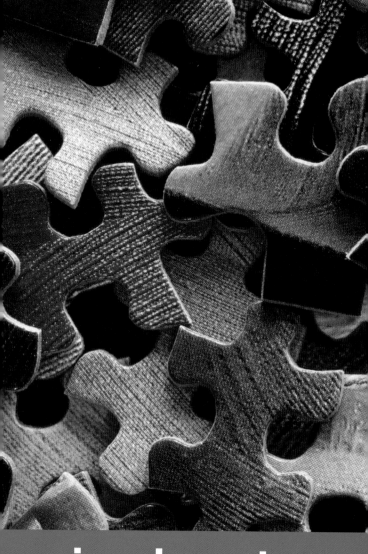

simple extras

FURTHER READING AND USEFUL CONTACTS

■ *BESTMEDICINE Lipid Disorders* (2005)
240pp, ISBN: 1-905064-90-X, £12.95
www.bestmedicine.com

■ Joint British Guidelines on the prevention of cardiovascular heart disease in clinical practice
New guidelines in press.

USEFUL CONTACTS

■ **Action on Smoking and Health**
Tel: 020 7739 5902
Website: *www.ash.org.uk*

■ **British Heart Foundation**
14 Fitzhardinge Street
London
W1H 6DH
Tel: 020 7935 0185
Website: *www.bhf.org.uk*
Heart information line: 08450 70 80 70

■ **British Nutrition Foundation**
High Holborn House
52–54 High Holborn
London
WC1V 6RQ
Tel: 020 7404 6504
Email: *postbox@nutrition.org.uk*
Website: *www.nutrition.org.uk*

■ **Diabetes UK**
Macleod House
10 Parkway
London
NW1 7AA
Tel: 020 7424 1000
Email: *info@diabetes.org.uk*
Website: *www.diabetes.org.uk*

■ **Food Standards Agency**
Aviation House
125 Kingsway
London
WC2B 6NH
Tel: 020 7276 8000
Website: *www.foodstandards.gov.uk*

■ **HEART UK**
7 North Road
Maidenhead
Berkshire
SL6 1PE
Tel: 01628 628 638
Website: *www.heartuk.org.uk*
Email: *ask@heartuk.org.uk*

■ **National Heart Forum**
Tavistock House South
Tavistock Square
London
WC1H 9LG.
Tel: 020 7383 7638
Website: *www.heartforum.org.uk*
Email: *webenquiry@heartforum.org.uk*

■ **NHS Direct**
www.nhsdirect.nhs.uk

■ **NHS Smoking Adviceline**: 0800 1690169

■ **The Patients Association**
PO Box 935
Harrow
Middlesex
HA1 3YJ
Helpline 0845 6084455
Tel: 020 8423 9111
Website: *www.patients-association.com*

■ **Stroke Association**
240 City Road
London
EC1V 2PR
Tel: 020 7566 0300
Website: *www.stroke.org.uk*
Email: *info@stroke.org.uk*
National Stroke Helpline: 0845 30 33 100

■ **Weightwatchers**
3rd Floor North Wing
Hines Meadow
St Cloud Way
Maidenhead
Berks
SL6 8XB
Email: *uk.help@weightwatchers.co.uk*
Website: *www.weightwatchers.co.uk*

DIETARY ADVICE TO HELP LOWER YOUR CHOLESTEROL (HEART UK)

BREAD, OTHER CEREALS AND POTATOES

Aim to base all meals on a good sized serving from this group. Have bread or bread products as healthy snacks.

Best choice – Wholegrain varieties of bread, chapatti without fat, pitta bread, flour tortillas, pasta, rice, basmati rice, noodles, wholegrain breakfast cereals, oats, couscous, potatoes, sweet potatoes, yam and plantain.

Occasionally (2–3 times/week) – Naan bread, reduced fat oven chips (with less than 5% fat), roast potatoes.

Best avoided! – Garlic bread, croissant, waffles, parathas, puris, samosas, pakoras, pilau, biryani and fried rice, sugar-coated breakfast cereals, deep-fried chips.

FRUIT AND VEGETABLES

Eat plenty; at least five or more portions everyday.

Best choice – Fresh, frozen, fruit and vegetables 100% juice, dried fruit, canned fruit in natural juice, vegetables canned in water, homemade vegetable based soups.

Occasionally (2–3 times/week) – Canned fruit in syrup (drain the syrup), reduced-fat coleslaw.

Best avoided! – Coleslaw, vegetables fried in batter (e.g. onion rings).

MEAT

Eat a moderate amount (1–2 portions a day). Vary by choosing low-fat meat, 2–3 times a week. On the other days choose fish or non-meat alternatives.

Best choice – Lean pork, ham, lamb, beef, extra lean minced beef, liver and kidney, chicken and turkey without skin, veal, venison, rabbit, game.

Occasionally (2–3 times/week) – Lean bacon, low-fat sausages, chicken breast in breadcrumbs, burgers, meatballs. Read the labels, find the lowest fat version.

Best avoided! – Fatty cuts of meat (belly pork, breast of lamb, duck, goose), frankfurters, streaky bacon, sausages and sausage rolls, pies, pasties, pork pies, chicken nuggets and kievs.

FISH

Try to eat fish at least twice a week, including one portion of oily fish. A portion of fish (or meat) is an amount the size of a pack of playing cards.

Best choice – All fish – cod, plaice, sole, whiting, canned tuna and shellfish. Oily fish – (fresh and canned) mackerel, sardines, pilchards, salmon, trout, herrings and fresh tuna.

Occasionally (2–3 times/week) – Canned fish in oil (drain oil), fried fish in batter (remove batter), fish fingers, fish cakes.

Best avoided! – Fish in rich creamy or cheesy sauces, hollandaise, lobster sauce, seafood cocktail sauce.

EGGS

A portion of eggs is 2 eggs.

Best choice – 3–4 per week – boiled, scrambled, poached without fat.

Occasionally (2–3 times/week) – Fried eggs and omelettes with minimal cooking fat.

Best avoided! – Quiche, scotch eggs.

NUTS AND SEEDS

A portion of nuts and seeds is 2 tablespoons.

Best choice – All nuts especially almonds, walnuts, linseed (flaxseed) pumpkin, sesame, sunflower seeds, nut/seed butters.

Occasionally (2–3 times/week) – Reduced-fat coconut milk.

Best avoided! – Coconut, coconut cream, roasted nuts in oil and salt, nut and seed butters with hydrogenated oils, palm oil.

BEANS, PEAS AND LENTILS, SOYA, TOFU AND QUORN

A portion of cooked beans, peas and lentils is 4 cooked tablespoons.

Best choice – Baked beans, sweetcorn, kidney beans, chick peas, lentils, peas. Rinse if canned in salt/sugar. Soya mince, soya beans, tofu, quorn sausages/burgers etc.

Occasionally (2–3 times/week) – Vegetarian sausages.

MILK AND MILK ALTERNATIVES

Aim to have 2–3 portions a day in drinks or in meals/snacks. A portion is a medium glass of milk (200 mL).

Best choice – Skimmed, semi-skimmed milk, semi-skimmed milk with plant sterols, soya milk (with added calcium and vitamins).

Occasionally (2–3 times/week) – Reduced-fat evaporated milk.

Best avoided! – Full-fat milk, sheep's, goat's milk, evaporated or condensed milk.

YOGURTS AND ALTERNATIVES

A portion is a small pot of yogurt or light fromage frais (150 g).

Best choice – Low-fat natural, fruit and diet yogurts, yogurts and mini-yogurt drinks with plant stanols/sterols, soya yogurts.

Occasionally (2–3 times/week) – Greek half-fat yogurt, whole milk yogurt.

Best avoided! – Greek yogurt, thick and creamy yogurt.

CHEESES

A portion is a matchbox of medium fat cheese (40 g) or 1/2 matchbox of high-fat cheese (20 g) or 2 small matchboxes of 'light' cheese spread (80 g) or a large pot of cottage cheese (200 g).

Best choice – Low-fat cheese e.g. cottage, curd cheese, quark, ricotta, half-fat Edam, 'extra light' cheese spread.

Occasionally (2–3 times/week) – Medium fat cheese e.g. half-fat Cheddar, Edam, Brie, camembert, soft goat's cheese, mozzarella, feta, 'light' cheese spread, paneer.

Best avoided! – High-fat cheese e.g. cream cheese, mascarpone, stilton, Cheddar type cheeses, vegetarian Cheddar, Gouda, parmesan, full-fat cheese spread, fried paneer.

FAT SPREADS

Best choice – Low fat unsaturated fat spreads, spreads with plant stanols/sterols.

Occasionally (2–3 times/week) – Spreads made from unsaturated oils.

Best avoided! – Butter, lard, suet, dripping, ghee, hard margarines, spreads with greater than 1% 'trans' fats – check label.

OILS

Use as little oil as possible, measure don't pour! Spray oil.

Best choice – Monounsaturated or polyunsaturated oils – olive, rapeseed, (most vegetable oil is made from rapeseed oil – check label) sunflower, soya, corn.

Best avoided! – Hydrogenated or partially hydrogenated vegetable oil (a source of 'trans' fats), oils which have been reheated several times.

CREAM AND CREAM ALTERNATIVES

Best choice – Virtually fat-free fromage frais.

Occasionally (2–3 times/week) – Half-cream, half-fat crème fraiche, fromage frais.

Best avoided! – Clotted, double, whipping, soured, single cream, crème fraiche.

DRESSINGS, SAUCES AND GRAVIES

Best choice – Use lemon juice, vinegar, herbs, yogurt etc. for salad dressings, thicken sauces and gravy with flour. Use low salt stock.

Occasionally (2–3 times/week) – Low-calorie salad creams and mayonnaise.

Best avoided! – Salad creams, mayonnaise, rich sauces made with cream or roux.

BISCUITS, CAKES, PASTRIES AND DESSERTS

Best choice – Plain biscuits, tea cakes, crumpets, malt bread, fruit salads, sorbet, sugar-free jelly.

Occasionally (2–3 times/week) – Home-made cakes and puddings using best choice ingredients, fruit-based puddings, ice cream, meringue.

Best avoided! – Cakes, pastries, pies, steamed puddings, trifle, doughnuts, cheesecake, cream, chocolate biscuits, shortbread.

SWEETS, CHOCOLATE AND PRESERVES

Best choice – Jams, honey, marmalade, sweeteners.

Occasionally (2–3 times/week) – Boiled sweets, mints, fruit gums.

Best avoided! – Chocolate, fudge, toffees, sugar, Indian sweets.

SAVOURY SNACKS

Best choice – Breadsticks, plain popcorn, unsalted nuts and seeds, dried fruit, thin-based pizzas.

Occasionally (2–3 times/week) – Low-fat crisps, reduced-fat hummus.

Best avoided! – Crisps, cheese snacks, Bombay mix, pizzas with too much cheese.

FLAVOURINGS

Best choice – Pepper, herbs, spices, lemon juice, garlic etc., chutney and pickles made without oil.

Occasionally (2–3 times/week) – Reduced-salt soy sauce.

Best avoided! – Salt, garlic salt, celery salt, soy sauce, oily pickles.

DRINKS

Drink 1.5–2 litres of fluid per day.

Best choice – Tap, mineral, soda water, fruit juice, tea, coffee with low-fat milks.

Occasionally (2–3 times/week) – Sugar-free squash, diet fizzy drinks, alcohol.

Best avoided! – Fruit squash, fizzy drinks.

LABELLING

Ready meals and foods you eat in large amounts look at the amounts per serving. For snacks and foods you eat in small amounts, look at the 'per 100 g' information.

A little is – 3 g of fat; 1 g of saturates, 0.1 g of sodium, or 0.25 g of salt.

A lot is - 20 g of fat, 5 g of saturates, 0.5 g of sodium, or 1.25 g of salt.

The original version of this table can be found at www.heartuk.org.uk

NOTES

_____

_____

_____

_____

_____

_____

_____

_____

_____

_____

_____

_____

_____

_____

_____